**PERGAMON INTERNATIONA**
of Science, Technology, Engineering an
*The 1000-volume original paperback library in*
*industrial training and the enjoyment (*
Publisher: Robert Maxwell, M.C.

# INTRODUCTION TO DISLOCATIONS
## Second Edition

International Series on

MATERIALS SCIENCE AND TECHNOLOGY

*Editor:* W. S. OWEN, D.Eng., Ph.D.

VOLUME 16

# Introduction to Dislocations

## SECOND EDITION

*by*

# DEREK HULL, Ph.D., C.Eng., D.Sc., F.I.M., F.P.R.I.

*Professor of Materials Engineering, University of Liverpool*

# PERGAMON PRESS

*Oxford · New York · Toronto · Sydney · Paris · Frankfurt*

| U.K. | Pergamon Press Ltd., Headington Hill Hall, Oxford OX3 0BW, England |
|---|---|
| U.S.A. | Pergamon Press Inc., Maxwell House, Fairview Park, Elmsford, New York 10523, U.S.A. |
| CANADA | Pergamon of Canada, Suite 104, 150 Consumers Road, Willowdale, Ontario M2 J1P9, Canada |
| AUSTRALIA | Pergamon Press (Aust.) Pty. Ltd., P.O. Box 544, Potts Point, N.S.W. 2011, Australia |
| FRANCE | Pergamon Press SARL, 24 rue des Ecoles, 75240 Paris, Cedex 05, France |
| FEDERAL REPUBLIC OF GERMANY | Pergamon Press GmbH, 6242 Kronberg-Taunus, Pferdstrasse 1, Federal Republic of Germany |

First edition 1965
Second edition 1975
Reprinted (with minor corrections) 1979

**Library of Congress Cataloging in Publication Data**

Hull, Derek.
Introduction to dislocations. 2nd edition
(International series on materials science and technology; v. 16)
Includes index.
1. Dislocations in crystals. I. Title.
QD945.H84 1975     548'.842     74-22359

ISBN 0 08 018129 5 hardcover
      0 08 018128 7 flexicover

*Printed in Great Britain by A. Wheaton & Co. Ltd., Exeter*

# Contents

# *Preface*

As I anticipated in the Preface to the First Edition, our basic knowledge of dislocations has remained unscathed in the last ten years. Much important research has been completed, but there is little which affects the underlying principles on which this introduction to dislocations is based. However, there have been changes and I welcome this opportunity to prepare a second edition.

There has been a continuing improvement in electron microscopy which has produced even more convincing evidence for dislocations and a vast amount of new data on dislocation distribution etc. Another technique which has developed rapidly is field ion microscopy which opens up a new dimension for studying the positions of atoms around dislocations. A powerful theoretical tool concerned with the same problem which has flourished since the first edition is computer simulation of crystal defects. Where appropriate these techniques have been referred to in the text and some half-tone illustrations have been changed.

One or two topics have been investigated exhaustively in the last ten years, notably the structure and properties of dislocations in body-centred cubic metals and their effect on the mechanical properties. The section on dislocations in other structures has been extended to take account of this work.

There has been the change to S.I. units. The transition has all the signs of the inevitable and to help the new generation of students this change has been made to the text. I offer my apologies to all those, like myself, who have got some feel for an e.V. and have now to move into the new world of aJ's.

Finally, my thanks to my 'dislocation' colleagues at Liverpool, Drs. Bacon, Bevis, Mordike and Noble who have made many helpful comments about the preparation of this new edition.

# Preface to the First Edition

ALTHOUGH the presence of dislocations in crystals was first proposed 30 years ago, it is only in the last 15 years that a general realisation of their importance has developed. Today, an understanding of dislocations is essential for all those concerned with the properties of crystalline materials. In the last 15 years the subject of dislocations has been transformed from an advanced research topic to one which is commonly taught at University undergraduate and technical school level. The subject has been richly served by two outstanding books, one by Professor A. H. Cottrell and the other by Dr. T. W. Read, both published 10 years ago, and by a tremendous amount of research literature. Although many aspects of the application of dislocation ideas are still in a state of flux a body of knowledge, based on theoretical analysis and experimental observation, has now been established which forms a basis for most of the ideas and theories which are proposed. Some fundamental dislocation problems remain to be solved but it seems unlikely that the ground work of the subject will be changed or modified appreciably, particularly at an introductory level.

In view of the importance of dislocations and the establishment of generally accepted principles, it seems appropriate to present an account of dislocations and their properties which can form an introduction to the understanding of many aspects of the properties of crystalline materials. Such is the intention of this book which is based on part of a one-year course on crystal defects and mechanical properties which I give to students of metallurgy. Parts of the course are given also in introductory courses on the properties of materials to physics and engineering students.

The method of approach in the book reflects the importance I attach to the necessity of the student achieving an intimate understanding of the three-dimensional geometry of dislocations in crystals. Once this is mastered, a qualitative appreciation of most ideas relating to dislocations can be assimilated.

The book is an account of the geometry, properties and behaviour of dislocations in crystals. The subject is developed from first principles so that the approach is applicable to all crystalline materials. In the first part the basic features of the geometry, movement and elastic properties of dislocations are described along with an account of the methods of observing and studying dislocations. This is followed by a description of the more detailed features of dislocations in specific structures; face-centred cubic, hexagonal close-packed, body-centred cubic, ionic, layer and superlattice structures. Two chapters are devoted to the basic properties of dislocations associated with their movement, such as intersections with other dislocations, jogs and multiplication of dislocations. Another chapter describes the geometry and properties of arrays of dislocations. Finally, the interaction between dislocations and imperfections in crystals, e.g. impurities, point defects, and other dislocations, is described and related to the stress required to move dislocations through a crystal containing such imperfections.

As far as possible the book is written in a form appropriate for an undergraduate course up to a final honours year level. Some of the material is probably beyond the normal honours year standard, but I consider that this is advisable in view of the need to familiarise the student with the next step as an aid to understanding the preceding steps. Less extensive courses than the honours standard can be developed readily from the first four chapters and parts of the other chapters.

Although not normally recommended in a student textbook, I have included a fairly extensive bibliography at the end of each chapter. The books and research papers which are listed were chosen carefully, and it is intended that they should be used by those who wish to take the subject one step further. They introduce also many of the more speculative aspects of the subject, and demonstrate the way dislocation theory is applied in practice. To help the student make a judicious choice, from the references given, the title of the work is included in addition to the reference source.

In attempting to collect together the available information on dislocations, it is inevitable that I should rely almost entirely on the published and unpublished work of others. I have been influenced particularly by the books by Cottrell and Read already referred to. Much of my outlook and knowledge of dislocations was developed and stimulated in a period of $3\frac{1}{2}$ years during which I carried out research in the basic irradiation group at Harwell. The group was led by Professor A. H. Cottrell, and included Drs. M. A. Adams, R. S. Barnes and M. J. Makin, and Professors R. E. Smallman and M. J. Thompson. My thanks are due to these friends for their stimulating company. I hope that I have given due recognition to all who have, by publishing their work, contributed to the contents of this book.

I have benefited greatly from the company of Professor W. S. Owen who kindly read through the manuscript and made many valuable suggestions. I should like also to thank Mr. I. L. Mogford and Mr. R. D. Garwood who read the manuscript in full, and many friends at Liverpool who read sections of the book and in so doing contributed to its final form.

A book of this kind would be impossible were it not for the many illustrations which are available. I am grateful to all authors and publishers who have freely given me permission to use their material. Specific acknowledgement is given in the captions. I am particularly grateful to many friends who have sent me copies from the original negatives of their photographs.

DEREK HULL

CHAPTER 1

# Defects in Crystals

## 1.1 Crystalline Materials

Metals and most non-metallic solids are crystalline, i.e. the constituent atoms are arranged in a pattern that repeats itself periodically in three dimensions. The actual arrangement of the atoms is called the *crystal structure*. The crystal structures of most pure metals are simple; the three most common structures being the body-centred cubic, face-centred cubic and close-packed hexagonal structures which are described in section 1.2. In contrast, the structures of alloys and non-metallic compounds are often complex.

The arrangement of atoms in a crystal can be described with respect to a three-dimensional net of straight lines as in Fig. 1.1(a). The lines divide space into equal sized parallelepipeds and the intersections of the lines is called a *space lattice*. Every point of a space lattice has identical surroundings. In simple structures the space lattice is usually constructed so that the lattice points correspond to atomic positions in the crystal, but it is not essential that every atomic site corresponds with a lattice site. Each parallelepiped is called a *unit cell* and the crystal is constructed by stacking identical unit cells face to face in perfect alignment in three dimensions.

The positions of the *planes*, *directions* and *point sites* in a lattice are described by reference to the unit cell and the three principal axes $x$, $y$ and $z$ (Fig. 1.1(b)). The cell dimensions $OA = a$, $OB = b$ and $OC = c$ are the lattice parameters, and these along with the angles $\angle BOC = \alpha$,

1

$\angle\ COA = \beta$ and $\angle\ AOB = \gamma$ completely define the size and shape of the cell. For simplicity the discussion will be restricted to cubic and hexagonal crystal structures. In cubic crystals $a = b = c$ and $\alpha = \beta = \gamma = 90°$, and the definition of planes and directions is straightforward. In hexagonal crystals a slightly more complicated approach is used and this is described in section 1.2.

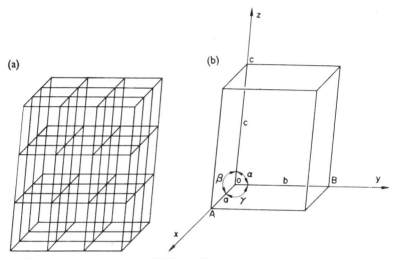

FIG. 1.1. (a) A space lattice. (b) Unit cell showing positions of principal axes.

Any *plane A'B'C'* in Fig. 1.2 can be defined by the intercepts $OA'$, $OB'$ and $OC'$ with the three principal axes. The usual notation (Miller indices) is to take the reciprocals of the ratios of the intercepts to the corresponding unit cell dimensions. Thus $A'B'C'$ is given by

$$\left(\frac{OA}{OA'}, \frac{OB}{OB'}, \frac{OC}{OC'}\right)$$

and the numbers are then reduced to the three smallest integers in these ratios.

Thus from Fig. 1.2 $OA' = 2a$, $OB' = 3a$, and $OC' = 3a$ the Miller indices of the $A'B'C'$ plane are (322). A plane with intercepts

$OA$, $OB$, and $OC$ is a

$$\left(\frac{OA}{OA}, \frac{OB}{OB}, \frac{OC}{OC}\right)$$

or

$$\left(\frac{a}{a}, \frac{a}{a}, \frac{a}{a}\right)$$

plane, namely (111). Similarly, a plane $DFBA$ in Fig. 1.3 is

$$\left(\frac{a}{a}, \frac{a}{a}, \frac{a}{\infty}\right)$$

or (110), a plane $DEGA$ is

$$\left(\frac{a}{a}, \frac{a}{\infty}, \frac{a}{\infty}\right)$$

or (100), and a plane $AB'C'$ in Fig. 1.2 is

$$\left(\frac{a}{a}, \frac{a}{3a}, \frac{a}{3a}\right)$$

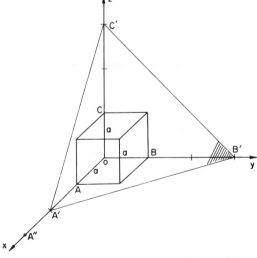

FIG. 1.2. Cubic cell illustrating method of describing positions of planes.

or (311). In determining the indices of any plane it is most convenient to identify the plane of lattice points parallel to the plane which is closest to the origin $O$ and intersects the principal axis close to the origin. Thus plane $A''B'C'$ in Fig. 1.2 is parallel to $ABC$ and it is clear that the indices are (111). Using this approach it will be seen that the planes $ABC$, $ABE$, $CEA$ and $CEB$ in Fig. 1.3 are (111), (11$\bar{1}$), (1$\bar{1}$1), and ($\bar{1}$11) respectively and constitute a group of planes of the same type described collectively by {111}. The minus sign above an index indicates that the plane cuts the axis on the negative side of the origin.

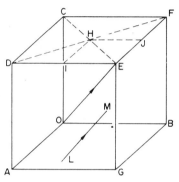

Fig. 1.3. Cubic cell illustrating the method of describing directions and point sites

Any *direction LM* in Fig. 1.3 is described by the line parallel to $LM$ through the origin, $OE$. The direction is given by the three smallest integers in the ratios of the lengths of $OE$ resolved along the three principal axes, namely $OA$, $OB$ and $OC$, as a fraction of the dimensions of the unit cell. Thus, if the unit cell is given by $OA$, $OB$ and $OC$ the direction $LM$ is

$$\left[\frac{OA}{OA}, \frac{OB}{OB}, \frac{OC}{OC}\right]$$

or

$$\left[\frac{a}{a}, \frac{a}{a}, \frac{a}{a}\right]$$

or [111]. Square brackets are used for directions. The directions *CG*, *AF*, *DB* and *EO* are [11$\bar{1}$], [$\bar{1}$11], [$\bar{1}$1$\bar{1}$] and [$\bar{1}$1$\bar{1}$] respectively and are a group of directions of the same type described collectively by $\langle 111 \rangle$. Similarly, direction *CE* is

or [110], direction *AG* is

$$\left[\frac{a}{a}, \frac{a}{a}, \frac{O}{a}\right]$$

$$\left[\frac{O}{a}, \frac{a}{a}, \frac{O}{a}\right]$$

or [010] and direction *GH* is

$$\left[\frac{-a/2}{a}, \frac{-a/2}{a}, \frac{a}{a}\right]$$

or [$\bar{1}\bar{1}$2].

In cubic crystals the Miller indices of a plane are the same as the indices of the direction normal to that plane. Thus in Fig. 1.3 the indices of the plane *EFBG* are (010) and the indices of the direction *AG* which is normal to *EFBG* are [010]. Similary, direction *OE* [111] is normal to plane *CBA* (111).

Any *point* in a crystal is described by the fractional displacements of the point from the three principal axes relative to the dimensions of the unit cell. The centre of the cell in Fig. 1.3 is $\frac{1}{2}, \frac{1}{2}, \frac{1}{2}$, and the points *F*, *E*, *H* and *I* are 0, 1, 1;    1, 1, 1;   $\frac{1}{2}, \frac{1}{2}, 1$; and 1, $\frac{1}{2}$, 1 respectively.

## 1.2 Simple Crystal Structures

In this section the atoms are considered as hard spheres which vary in size from element to element. From the hard sphere model the parameters of the unit cell can be described directly in terms of the radius of the sphere, $r$. In the diagrams illustrating the crystal structures the atoms are shown as small circles in the three-dimensional drawings and as large circles representing the full hard sphere sizes in the two-dimensional diagrams. It will be shown that many crystal structures can be described as a stack of atom layers in which the arrangement of atoms in each layer is identical. The positions of the atoms in layers above and below the layer, represented by the plane of the diagram, are shown by small shaded circles in the two-dimensional diagrams. The order or sequence of the atom layers in the stack, i.e. the *stacking sequence*, is referred to by fixing one layer as an *A* layer and all other layers with atoms in identical positions as *A* layers also. Layers of atoms in other positions in the stack are referred to as *B*, *C*, *D* layers, etc.

In the *simple cubic structure*, illustrated in Fig. 1.4, the atoms are situated at the corners of the unit cell. Figures 1.4(b) and (c) show

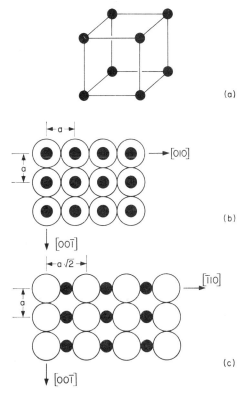

FIG. 1.4. Simple cubic structure: (a) unit cell, (b) arrangement of atoms in (100) layers, (c) arrangements of atoms in (110) layers.

the arrangements of atoms in the (100) and (110) planes respectively. The atoms touch along ⟨001⟩ directions and therefore the lattice parameter $a$ is twice the atomic radius $r$, ($a = 2r$). The atoms in adjacent (100) planes are in identical atomic sites relative to the direction normal to this plane so that the stacking sequence of (100) planes is $AAA...$ The atoms in adjacent (110) planes are displaced $\frac{1}{2}a\sqrt{2}$ along [$\bar{1}$10] relative to each other and the spacing of atoms along

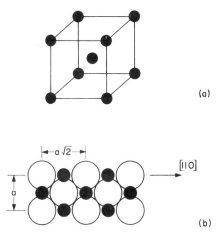

(a)

(b)

FIG. 1.5. Body-centred cubic structures (a) unit cell, (b) arrangement of atoms in (110) layers.

[$\bar{1}$10] is $a\sqrt{2}$. It follows that alternate planes have atoms in the same atomic sites relative to the direction normal to (110) and the stacking sequence of (110) planes is $ABABAB...$ The spacing between successive (110) planes is $\frac{1}{2}a\sqrt{2}$.

In the *body-centred cubic structure* (Fig. 1.5) the atoms are situated at the corners of the unit cell and at the centre site $\frac{1}{2}, \frac{1}{2}, \frac{1}{2}$. The atoms touch along ⟨111⟩ directions and this is referred to as the *close-packed direction*. The lattice parameter $a = 4r/\sqrt{3}$ and the spacing of atoms along ⟨110⟩ directions is $a\sqrt{2}$. The stacking sequence of {100} and {110} planes is $ABABAB...$ (Fig. 1.5(b)). There is particular interest in the stacking of {112} type planes. Figure 1.6 shows two body-centred cubic cells and the positions of a set of ($\bar{1}1\bar{2}$) planes. Since, for cubic structures the indices of directions normal to a set of planes are the same as those of the plane a plan of the ($\bar{1}1\bar{2}$) planes viewed along [$\bar{1}1\bar{2}$] will represent the arrangement of atoms in succes-

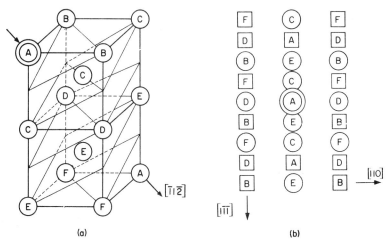

(a)                                    (b)

FIG. 1.6. Diagrammatic representation of the stacking sequence of ($\bar{1}1\bar{2}$) layers in a body-centred cubic structure: (a) two unit cells showing positions of ($\bar{1}1\bar{2}$) planes, (b) position of atoms in ($\bar{1}1\bar{2}$) layers; the atom sites marked by circles are contained in the two cells shown in (a), those marked by squares are not contained in (a).

sive layers. From the diagrams it is seen that the stacking sequence of the ($\bar{1}1\bar{2}$) planes is *ABCDEFAB*..., and the spacing between the planes is $a/\sqrt{6}$.

In the *face-centred cubic structure*, shown in Fig. 1.7, the atoms are situated at the corners of the unit cell and at the centres of all the cube faces in sites of the type $0, \frac{1}{2}, \frac{1}{2}$. The atoms touch along the $\langle 011 \rangle$ close-packed directions. The lattice parameter $a = 2r\sqrt{2}$. The stacking sequence of $\{100\}$ and $\{110\}$ planes is *ABABAB*..., and the stacking sequence of (111) planes is *ABCABC*... The latter is of considerable importance and is illustrated in Figs. 1.7(b) and (c). The atoms in the (111) planes are in the most close-packed arrangement possible and contain three close-packed directions 60° apart.

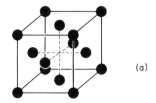

(a)

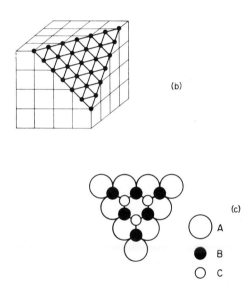

(b)

(c)

◯ A

● B

◯ C

F<small>IG</small>. 1.7. Face-centred cubic structure: (a) unit cell, (b) arrangement of atoms in a (111) close-packed plane, (c) stacking sequence of (111) planes.

The *close-packed hexagonal structure* is more complex than the cubic structures but can be described very simply with reference to the stacking sequence. The lattice is formed by an *ABABAB*... sequence of the close-packed planes as in the (111) plane of the face-centred cubic lattice. In Fig. 1.8(a) an hexagonal lattice has been outlined in an *ABA* stack. The unit cell is outlined more heavily. Atoms are situated at the corners of the unit cell and at $\frac{2}{3}, \frac{1}{3}, \frac{1}{2}$. A face-centred cubic structure can be obtained from a close-packed hexagonal structure by changing the stacking sequence from *ABABAB...* to *ABCABC...* For a hard sphere model the ratio of the length of the *c* and *a* axes (axial ratio) of the hexagonal structure is 1·633. In practice, the axial ratio varies between 1·57 and 1·89 in close-packed hexagonal

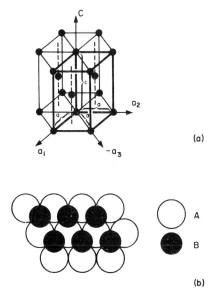

(a)

(b)

FIG. 1.8. Close-packed hexagonal structure: (a) hexagonal cell formed by an *ABA* sequence of close-packed planes, the unit cell is marked by the heavy lines, (b) *ABAB...* stacking sequence.

metals. The variations arise because the hard sphere model gives only an approximate value of the interatomic distances and requires modification depending on the electronic structure of the atoms.

The planes and directions in the hexagonal lattice are normally referred to the four axes $a_1$, $a_2$, $a_3$ and $c$ indicated in Fig. 1.8(a). When the reciprocal intercepts of a plane on all four axes are found and reduced to the smallest integers, the indices are of the type $(h, k, i, l)$, and the first three indices are related by

$$i = -(h+k). \tag{1.1}$$

Equivalent planes are obtained by interchanging the position and sign of the first three indices. A number of planes in the hexagonal lattice have been given specific names. For example:

Basal plane                                  (0001)

Prism plane (type I)                 $(1\bar{1}00)$    $(\bar{1}100)$, etc.

Prism plane (type II)              $(11\bar{2}0)$    $(\bar{2}110)$, etc.

Pyramidal plane (type I) first order    $(10\bar{1}1)$    $(\bar{1}011)$, etc.

Pyramidal plane (type II) first order   $(11\bar{2}1)$    $(\bar{1}\bar{1}21)$, etc.

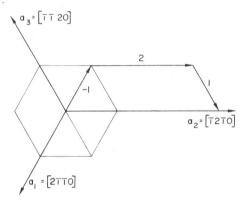

FIG. 1.9. Determination of direction indices in a the basal plane of an hexagonal crystal.

Some of these planes are indicated in Fig. 6.3. Direction indices in hexagonal structures are translations parallel to the four axes that cause the motion in the required direction. The numbers must be reduced to the smallest integers and chosen so that the third index is the negative of the sum of the first two. To satisfy this condition the directions along axes $a_1$, $a_2$ and $a_3$ are of the type $[\bar{1}2\bar{1}0]$ as illustrated in Fig. 1.9.

### 1.3 Perfect Crystals

Large crystals can be built up from a three-dimensional array of atoms producing a perfect structure in which every atom site is filled and there is no disturbance in the regular arrangement of atom planes. The chemical and physical properties of this perfect or ideal crystal depend on the structure of the atoms and the nature of the atomic binding.

All real crystals contain *imperfections* which may be *point*, *line*, *surface* or *volume* defects, and which disturb locally the regular arrangement of the atoms. Before describing these defects in detail some qualitative examples are considered which emphasise the important role they play in determining the properties of crystals. The large *electrical conductivity of metals* can be attributed to the ease of flow of "free" electrons through the lattice. Any electrical resistance is due to the scattering of electrons by the lattice. In a perfect crystal at a temperature above 0 K scattering occurs because all the atoms and ions are in a state of continual vibration about their equilibrium positions and this modifies the periodic arrangement. The amplitude of the vibrations increases with increasing temperature and the scattering of electrons, and therefore the electrical resistivity, increases also. The theory of scattering due to such vibrations predicts that at very low temperatures

$$\varrho_1 \propto T^5, \qquad (1.2)$$

where $\varrho_1$ is the electrical resistivity and $T$ is the absolute temperature, and that at high temperatures

$$\varrho_1 \propto T. \qquad (1.3)$$

In practice it is found that there is a second component $\varrho_2$ in the electrical resistivity which is approximately independent of temperature. When $\varrho_2$ is subtracted from the total resistivity, i.e. $\varrho - \varrho_2 = \varrho_1$, $\varrho_1$ is found to be in good agreement with equations (1.2) and (1.3) for many metals. Experiments show that $\varrho_2$, which predominates at low temperatures, is sensitive to impurity content, plastic deformation, energetic radiations and quenching. All these introduce crystal defects which cause scattering of the electrons due to local changes in the periodic arrangement of the atoms. Where reliable estimates or measurements of the change in $\varrho_2$ per defect can be made, electrical resistivity is a sensitive method of measuring the concentration of such defects.

One of the successes of the theory of crystal defects, which contributed appreciably to the universal acceptance of the existence of line defects called *dislocations* in crystals, was the reconciliation of classical *theory of crystal growth* with the experimental observations of growth rates. Consider a perfect crystal having irregular facets growing in a supersaturated vapour. At a low degree of supersaturation growth occurs by the deposition of atoms on the irregular or imperfect regions of the crystal. The preferential deposition in imperfect regions results in the formation of more perfect faces consisting of close-packed arrays of atoms. Further growth then requires the nucleation of a new layer of atoms on a smooth face. This is a much more difficult process and nucleation theory predicts that for growth to occur at the observed rates a degree of supersaturation of approximately 50 per cent would be required. This is contrary to many experimental observations which show that growth occurs readily at a supersaturation of only 1 per cent. The difficulty was resolved when it was demonstrated that the presence of dislocations in the crystal during growth could result in the formation of steps on the crystal faces which are not removed by preferential deposition, as in a perfect crystal. These steps provided sites for deposition and thus eliminated the difficult nucleation process.

*Plastic deformation of a perfect* crystal can occur by the sliding of one set of atoms in a plane over the atoms in an adjacent plane. This is a co-operative movement of all the atoms in a plane from one position of perfect registry to the neighbouring position. The shear stress required for this process was first calculated by Frenkel. The situation is illustrated in Fig. 1.10. If it is assumed that there is a periodic shearing force required to move the top row of atoms across the bottom row which is given by the sinusoidal relation:

$$\tau = \frac{Gb}{2\pi a} \sin \frac{2\pi x}{b} \tag{1.4}$$

where $G$ is the shear modulus, $b$ the spacing between atoms in the direction of the shear stress, $a$ the spacing of the rows of atoms and $x$ the distance away from the low-energy equilibrium position, then the theoretical critical shear stress is

$$\tau_{th} = \frac{b}{a}\frac{G}{2\pi}.$$  (1.5)

Since $b \approx a$ the theoretical shear stress is only a small fraction of the shear modulus. Using a more realistic expression for the shearing force as a function of displacement a value of $\tau_{th} \approx G/30$ for copper, silver and gold has been obtained. Although these are approximate calculations they show that $\tau_{th}$ is many orders of magnitude greater than the observed values ($10^{-4}$ to $10^{-6}$ $G$) of the resolved shear stresses measured in real, well-annealed crystals. This striking difference between prediction and experiment was accounted for by the presence of dislocations. In recent years it has been possible to

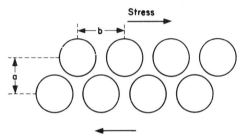

Fig. 1.10. Representation of atom positions used to estimate critical shear stress for slip.

produce crystals in the form of fibres with a small diameter, called whiskers, which have a very high degree of perfection. These whiskers are sometimes entirely free of dislocations and their strength is close to the theoretical strength.

These examples are sufficient to indicate that a knowledge of the structure of defects and their properties is essential to those who concern themselves with any aspect of the properties of materials. This book is concerned primarily with the line defects called *dislocations*. However, there is a very close relation between all the crystal defects and in the next section some of these defects are described.

## 1.4 Defects in Crystalline Materials

POINT DEFECTS

All the atoms in a perfect lattice are at specific atomic sites (ignoring the thermal vibrations referred to in section 1.3). In a pure metal two types of point defect are possible, namely a *vacant atomic site* or *vacancy*, and an *interstitial atom*. These defects are illustrated, for a simple cubic structure, in Fig. 1.11. The vacancy has been formed by the removal of an atom from an atomic site and the interstitial by the introduction of an atom into a non-atomic site at a $\frac{1}{2}, \frac{1}{2}, 0$ posi-

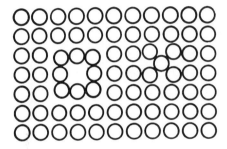

(a)                    (b)

FIG. 1.11. (a) Vacancy, (b) interstitial atom in an (001) plane of a simple cubic lattice.

tion. There is a considerable amount of experimental evidence that vacancies and interstitials can be produced in materials by plastic deformation and high energy particle irradiation, and that a high density of vacancies can be retained in a crystal by rapid quenching from a high temperature. The last effect arises because at all temperatures above 0 K there is a thermodynamically stable number of vacancies. The change in free energy $\Delta F$ associated with the introduction of $n$ vacancies in the lattice is

$$\Delta F = nU_v - T\Delta S \tag{1.6}$$

where $U_v$ is the energy of formation of one vacancy which is created by removing one atom from the lattice and placing it on the surface of the crystal, and $\Delta S$ is the change in the entropy of the crystal. $nU_v$ represents a considerable positive energy but this is offset by an increase in the configurational entropy due to the presence of the vacancies. The equilibrium fraction of vacancies corresponding to a condition of minimum free energy is

$$n_{eq} = n_t \exp\left(-\frac{U_v}{kT}\right) \tag{1.7}$$

where $n_t$ is the total number of atomic sites and $k$ is Boltzmann's constant. A typical value of $U_v$ for copper is 1·1 aJ (0·7 eV) so that at 1250 K the fraction of sites vacant $n_{eq}/n_t$ is $\sim 10^{-3}$, and at 300 K $n_{eq}/n_t$ is $\sim 10^{-12}$. The rate at which vacancies move from point to point in the lattice decreases exponentially with decreasing temperature and consequently in many metals it is possible to retain the high temperature concentration at room temperature by quenching from the equilibrating temperature.

Impurity atoms in a pure metal can also be considered as point defects and they play a very important role in the physical and mechanical properties of all materials. Impurity atoms can take up two different types of site, as illustrated in Fig. 1.12, (a) *substitutional*,

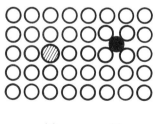

(a)          (b)

Fig. 1.12. (a) Substitutional impurity atom, (b) interstitial impurity atom.

in which an atom of the parent lattice lying in a lattice site is replaced by the impurity atom, and (b) *interstitial*, in which the impurity atom is at a non-atomic site similar to the interstitial atoms referred to above.

All the point defects mentioned produce a local distortion in the otherwise perfect lattice. The amount of distortion and hence the amount of additional energy in the lattice due to the defects depends on the amount of "space" between the atoms in the lattice and the "size" of the atoms introduced. Additional effects are important when the removal or addition of atoms changes the local electric charge in the lattice. This is relatively unimportant in crystals with metallic binding, but can be demonstrated particularly well in crystals in which the binding is ionic. The structure of sodium chloride is shown in Fig. 1.13. Each negatively charged chlorine ion is surrounded by

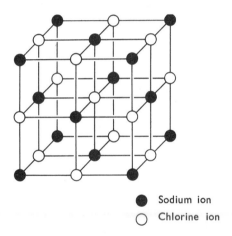

● Sodium ion
○ Chlorine ion

FIG. 1.13. Sodium chloride structure which consists of two interpenetrating face-centred cubic lattices of the two types of atom, with the corner of one located at the point $\frac{1}{2}$, 0 0 of the other.

six nearest neighbours of positively charged sodium ions and vice versa. The removal of a sodium or a chlorine ion produces a local positive or negative charge as well as a vacant lattice site. These are called *cation* and *anion* vacancies respectively. To conserve an overall neutral charge the vacancies must occur either (a) in pairs of opposite sign, *Schottky defects*, or (b) in association with interstitials of the same ion, *Frenkel defects*.

STACKING FAULTS

In section 1.2 it was emphasised that perfect lattices can be described as a stack of identical atom layers arranged in a regular sequence. A stacking fault is a *planar defect* and, as its name implies, it is a local region in the crystal where the regular sequence has been interrupted. Stacking faults are not expected in planes with *ABABAB* ... sequences in body-centred or face-centred cubic lattices because there is no alternative site for an *A* layer resting on a *B* layer. However, for *ABCABC* ... stacking of the close-packed lattices there are two possible positions of one layer resting on another. A close-packed layer of atoms resting on an *A* layer can rest equally well in either a *B* or a *C* position and geometrically there is no reason for the selection of a particular position. In a face-centred cubic

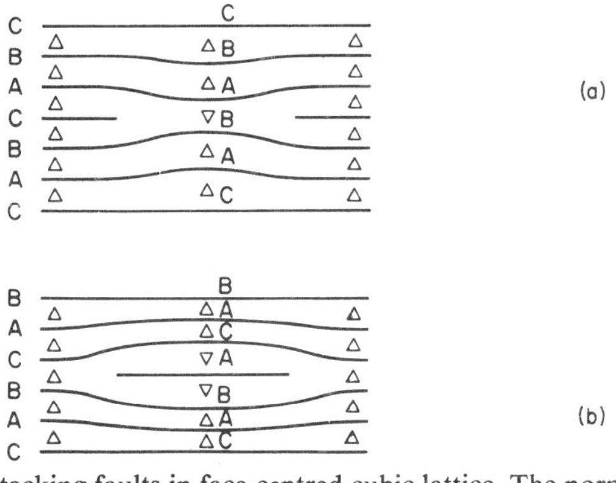

FIG. 1.14. Stacking faults in face-centred cubic lattice. The normal stacking sequence of (111) planes is denoted by *ABCA* ... Planes in normal relation to one another are separated by $\triangle$; those with a stacking error by $\triangledown$, (a) intrinsic stacking fault, (b) extrinsic stacking fault.

lattice two types of stacking fault are possible, referred to as *intrinsic* and *extrinsic*. These are best described by considering the change in sequence resulting from the removal or introduction of an extra layer. In Fig. 1.14(a) part of a *C* layer has been removed which results in a break in the stacking sequence. This is an *intrinsic fault* and it can be seen that the lattice patterns above and below the fault

plane are continuous right up to the fault plane. In Fig. 1.14(b) an
extra *A* layer has been introduced between a *B* and a *C* layer. There
are two breaks in the stacking sequence and it is referred to as an
*extrinsic fault*. The extra layer does not belong to the continuing
patterns of either the lattice above or below the fault. Stacking faults
have a characteristic energy per unit area called the *stacking fault
energy*. Because of the additional lattice discontinuity associated
with an extrinsic fault it is expected to have a higher stacking fault
energy than an intrinsic fault.

The stacking faults which occur in a close-packed hexagonal lattice
are described in Chapter 6.

DISLOCATIONS

The concept of a linear lattice imperfection called a dislocation
arose primarily from the study of plastic deformation processes in
crystalline materials. This approach is used in Chapter 3 and leads
to a good understanding of the nature of dislocations. At this stage
it will be sufficient to describe the basic geometry of an *edge* and a
*screw* dislocation and introduce the appropriate definitions and ter-
minology.

Figure 1.15(a) represents an elementary descriptive model of the
atomic arrangement and bonding in a simple cubic structure. For
convenience it is assumed that the bonds can be represented by flexible
springs between adjacent atoms. It must be emphasised that bonding
in real solids is complex and, in fact, the nature of the bonding
determines the fine detail of the arrangement of the atoms around
the dislocation. The model shows that the application of a shear
stress to the crystal lattice will produce an "elastic" distortion. The
arrangement of atoms around an edge dislocation can be simulated
by the following sequence of operations. Suppose that all the bonds
across the surface *ABCD* are broken and the faces of the crystal are
separated so that an extra plane of atoms can be inserted in the slot,
as illustrated in Fig. 1.15(b). The faces of the slot will have been
displaced by one atom spacing but the only large disturbance of the

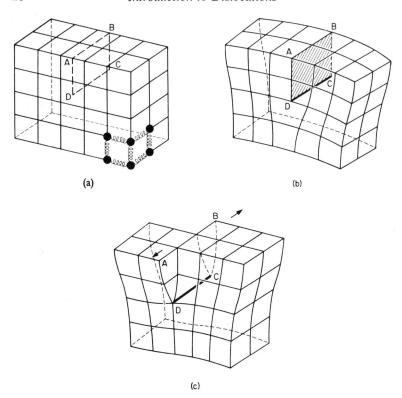

(a)

(b)

(c)

Fɪɢ. 1.15. (a) Model of a simple cubic lattice; the atoms are represented by hard spheres, and the bonds between atoms by springs, only a few of which are shown, (b) positive edge dislocation *DC* formed by inserting an extra half plane of atoms in *ABCD*; (c) left-handed screw dislocation *DC* formed by displacing the faces *ABCD* relative to each other in direction *AB*.

atoms from their normal positions is close to the line *DC*. This line *DC* is called a *positive edge dislocation* and is represented symbolically by ⊥. The introduction of the extra plane of atoms produces a small deflection of the lattice planes as well as the distorted region close to the dislocation line. A *negative edge dislocation* would be obtained by inserting the extra plane of atoms below plane *ABCD* and is represented by ⊤.

The arrangement of atoms round a screw dislocation can be simulated by displacing the crystal on one side of *ABCD* relative to the other side in the direction *AB* as in Fig. 1.15(c). Examination of this model shows that it can be described as a *single surface helicoid*, rather like a spiral staircase. Consider the line *AD*, fixed along *DC*, and rotate it in an anti-clockwise direction in the (100) plane of the crystal. After a rotation of 360° it has moved down one lattice spacing on an unbroken plane and it can continue to rotate moving through the crystal on the helicoidal surface. *DC* is a screw dislocation. Looking down the dislocation line, if the helix advances one plane when a *clockwise circuit* is made round it, it is referred to as a *right-handed screw* dislocation, and if the reverse is true it is *left-handed*.

It is important to realise that in both the edge and the screw dislocations described the registry of atoms across the interface *ABCD* is identical to that before the bonds were broken.

**Burgers vector and Burgers circuit.** The most useful definition of a dislocation is given in terms of the *Burgers circuit*. A Burgers circuit is any atom to atom path taken in a crystal containing dislocations which forms a closed loop. Such a path is illustrated in Fig. 1.16(a), i.e. *MNOPQ*. If the same atom to atom sequence is made in a dis-

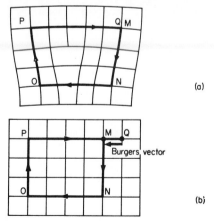

FIG. 1.16. (a) Burgers circuit round an edge dislocation, (b) the same circuit in a perfect crystal; the closure failure is the Burgers vector.

location free crystal and the circuit does not close then the first circuit, Fig. 1.16(a), must enclose one or more dislocations. The vector required to complete the circuit is called the *Burgers vector*. It is essential that the circuit in the real crystal passes entirely through "good" parts of the crystal. For simplicity consider the Burgers circuit to enclose one dislocation as in Fig. 1.16(a). The sequence of atom to atom movements in the perfect crystal is the same as for the circuit *MNOPQ* in Fig. 1.16(a). The closure failure *QM* is the Burgers vector and is at *right angles* to the dislocation line (cf. Fig. 1.15(b)). When the Burgers circuit is drawn round a screw dislocation (Fig. 1.17), again with a closed circuit in the crystal containing the disloca-

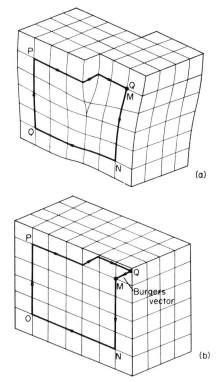

Fig. 1.17. (a) Burgers circuit round a screw dislocation; (b) the same circuit in a perfect crystal; the closure failure is the Burgers vector.

tion, the Burgers vector $QM$ is parallel to the dislocation line. This leads to two important rules:

(a) *The Burgers vector of an edge dislocation is normal to the line of the dislocation,*
(b) *The Burgers vector of a screw dislocation is parallel to the line of the dislocation.*

In the most general case (Chapter 3) the dislocation line lies at an arbitrary angle to its Burgers vector and the dislocation line has a *mixed* edge and screw character. However, *the Burgers vector of the dislocation is always the same and independent of the position of the dislocation.*

Since, by definition, the Burgers circuit is an atom to atom movement the closure failure must always be between two atom sites in the perfect crystal and will be a *lattice vector*. A dislocation defined in this way is a *perfect* or *unit dislocation*. A convenient notation has been adopted for describing the Burgers vector **b** of a dislocation, i.e. the magnitude and direction of the vector. For example, the lattice vector from the origin to the centre of a body-centred cubic cell is defined both in magnitude and direction by displacements of $a/2$ in the $x$-direction, $a/2$ in the $y$-direction and $a/2$ in the $z$-direction, and the notation used is $\mathbf{b} = \frac{1}{2}[111]$. The strength $b$ of the vector is

$$b = \sqrt{\left(\frac{a^2}{4} + \frac{a^2}{4} + \frac{a^2}{4}\right)} = \frac{a\sqrt{3}}{2}.$$ (1.8)

Dislocation lines can end at the surface of a crystal and at grain boundaries, but never inside a crystal. Thus, *dislocations must either form closed loops or branch into other dislocations.* When three or more dislocations meet at a point, or *node*, it is a necessary condition that the sum of the Burgers vectors equals zero. Consider the dislocation $\mathbf{b}_1$ (Fig. 1.18) which branches into two dislocations with Burgers vectors $\mathbf{b}_2$ and $\mathbf{b}_3$. A Burgers circuit has been drawn round each dislocation in the same sense, and it follows from the diagram that

$$\mathbf{b}_1 = \mathbf{b}_2 + \mathbf{b}_3$$ (1.9)

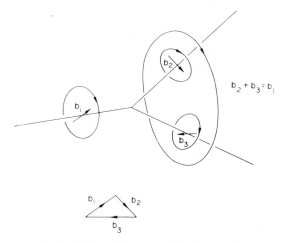

FIG. 1.18. Three dislocations forming a node.

The large circuit on the right-hand side of the diagram encloses two dislocations, but since is passes through the same good material as the $b_1$ circuit on the left-hand side the Burgers vector must be the same, i.e. $b_1$. It is more usual to define the Burgers circuits by making a clockwise circuit around each dislocation line looking outward from the nodal point. Then equation (1.9) becomes

$$b_1 + b_2 + b_3 = 0 \qquad (1.10)$$

or more generally

$$\sum_1^n b_i = 0. \qquad (1.11)$$

All crystals, apart from some whiskers, contain dislocations and in well-annealed crystals the dislocations are arranged in a rather ill-defined network, the *Frank net*, which is illustrated schematically in Fig. 1.19. The number of dislocations in a unit volume of crystal, *dislocation density* $N$, is defined as the total length of dislocation $l$ per unit volume, $N = l/V$ normally quoted in units of $cm^{-2}$. A less precise definition, but one which is usually more convenient to use, is the number of dislocations intersecting a unit area, again measured in units of cm$^{-2}$. In well-annealed metal crystals $N$ is usually between $10^6$ and $10^8$ cm$^{-2}$, but with very careful treatment, can be as low as

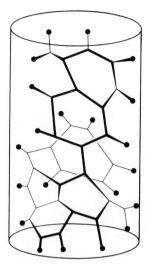

FIG. 1.19. Diagrammatic illustration of the arrangement of dislocations in a well annealed crystal; the Frank net. (From COTTRELL, *The Properties of Materials at High Rates of Strain*, Instn Mech. Eng., London, 1957.)

$10^2$ cm$^{-2}$. $N$ increases rapidly with plastic deformation and a typical value for a heavily cold rolled metal is about $5 \times 10^{11}$ cm$^{-2}$. $N$ is usually lower in non-metallic crystals than in metal crystals.

GRAIN BOUNDARIES

Crystalline solids usually consist of a large number of randomly oriented grains separated by grain boundaries. Each grain is a single crystal and contains the defects already described. When the mis-orientation between the grains is small the boundary consists of an array of dislocations and is called a *low angle boundary*, see Chapter 9. However, when the misorientation is large the atomic arrangement at the boundary is more complicated and varies significantly with the angle of misorientation. An easy way to visualise the atomic arrangement is to use bubble models (Fig. 1.20) in which a two-dimensional raft of equal sized bubbles floats on the surface of a liquid. Figure 1.20 shows a grain or "crystal" surrounded by grains

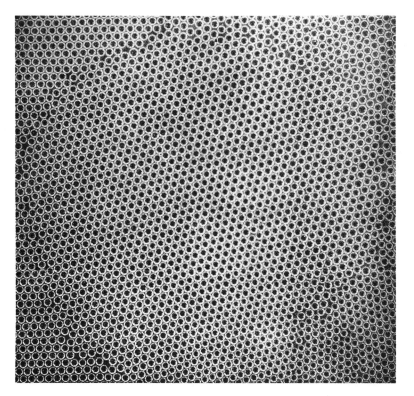

FIG. 1.20. Crystal grain simulated by a bubble raft. (From *Scientific American*, Sept. 1967.)

of different orientation. A notable feature of the boundary structure is that the region of disorder is very narrow being limited to one or two atoms on each side of the boundary. Bubble raft "dislocations" can also be seen in the bottom right-hand corner of Fig. 1.20.

TWIN BOUNDARIES

When adjacent parts of a crystal are regularly arranged such that one part is a mirror image of the other, the two parts are said to be twin related. The mirror plane is called the *composition plane* and

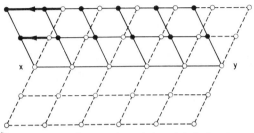

FIG. 1.21. Arrangement of atoms in a twin related structure; $x$–$y$ is the trace of the twin composition plane.

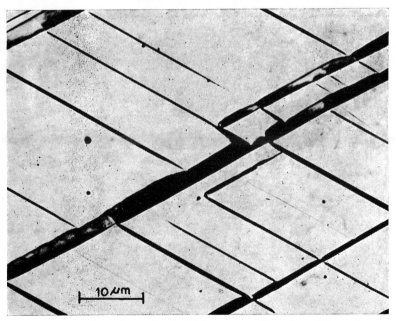

FIG. 1.22. Deformation twins in 3·25 per cent silicon iron. The surface at the twins is tilted so light is reflected in a different direction.

is illustrated in Fig. 1.21. The open circles represent the positions of the atoms before twinning and the black circles the positions after twinning. The atoms above $x$–$y$ are mirror images of the atoms below it and therefore $x$–$y$ represents the trace of the twin composition plane in the plane of the paper. Twinning can be represented as a homogeneous shear of the lattice parallel to the composition plane. The process differs from slip (Chapter 3) in which there is no rotation of the lattice. Twins are a common feature in annealed face-centred cubic metals which have a low stacking fault energy (annealing twins), but they are not restricted to these metals. Under suitable conditions twinning can be induced by plastic deformation (deformation twinning) and this is particularly important in body-centred cubic and close-packed hexagonal metals. When a growing twin meets a flat surface it will produce a well-defined tilt and this can readily be detected in an optical microscope. Figure 1.22 shows the tilts produced by deformation twins in a 3·25 per cent silicon iron crystal deformed at 20 K.

## Further Reading

CRYSTAL STRUCTURE

BARRETT, C. S. and MASSALSKI, T. B. (1966) *Structure of Metals*, McGraw-Hill.
BUERGER, M. J. (1963) *Elementary Crystallography*, Wiley.
CULLITY, B. D. (1959) *Elements of X-ray Diffraction*, Addison-Wesley.
KELLY, A. and GROVES, G. W. (1970) *Crystallography and Crystal Defects*, Longman.

ATOMIC STRUCTURE

HUME-ROTHERY, W. (1948) *Atomic Theory for Students of Metallurgy*, The Institute of Metals.
KITTEL, C. (1967) *Introduction to Solid State Physics*, Wiley.
WERT C. A. and THOMSON R. M. (1964) *Physics of Solids*, McGraw-Hill.

POINT DEFECTS

COTTERILL, R. M. K. DOYAMA, M., JACKSON, J. J. and MESHII, M. (Eds.) (1965) *Lattice Defects in Quenched Metals*, Academic Press.
DAMASK, A. C. and DIENES, G. J. (1963) *Point Defects in Metals*, Gordon & Breach.

DISLOCATIONS

COTTRELL, A. H. (1953) *Dislocations and Plastic Flow in Crystals*, Oxford University Press.
"Dislocations in solids" (1964) *Disc. Faraday Soc.* **38**.
FISHER, J. C., JOHNSTON, W. G., THOMPSON, R. and VREELAND, T. (1957) *Dislocations and Mechanical Properties of Crystals*, Wiley.
FRIEDEL, J. (1964) *Dislocations*, Pergamon Press.
GILMAN, J. J. (1969) *Micromechanics of Flow in Solids*, McGraw-Hill.
HIRTH, J. P. and LOTHE, J. (1968) *Theory of Dislocations*, McGraw-Hill.
KELLY, A. and GROVES, G. W. (1970) *Crystallography and Crystal Defects*, Longman.
NABARRO, F. R. N. (1967) *The Theory of Crystal Dislocations*, Oxford University Press.
READ, W. T. (1953) *Dislocations in Crystals*, McGraw-Hill.
SEEGER, A. (1955) "Theory of lattice imperfections", *Handbuch der Physik*, Vol. VII, part 1, p. 383, Springer-Verlag.
SEEGER, A. (1958) "Plasticity of crystals", *Handbuch der Physik*, Vol. VII, part II. p. 1, Springer-Verlag.
TAYLOR, G. I. (1934) "Mechanism of plastic deformation in crystals", *Proc. Roy, Soc.* A **145.** 362.
THOMAS, J. M. (1970) "The chemistry of deformed and imperfect crystals", *Endeavour*, **29,** 149.
WEERTMAN, J. and WEERTMAN, J. R. (1964) *Elementary Dislocation Theory*, Macmillan.

STACKING FAULTS AND TWINS

CHRISTIAN, J. W. and SWANN, P. R. (1963) "Stacking faults in metals and alloys" in *Alloying Effects on Concentrated Solid Solutions*. A.I.M.E.
HALL, E. O. (1954) *Twinning*, Butterworth & Co.
KLASSEN-NEKLYUDOVA, M. V. (BRADLEY, J. E. S. (trans.)) (1964) *Mechanical Twinning of Crystals*, Consultants Bureau.
REED-HILL, R. E. HIRTH, J. P. and ROGERS, H. C. (Eds.) (1965) *Deformation Twinning*, Gordon & Breach.

CHAPTER 2

# *Observation of Dislocations*

## 2.1 Introduction

A wide range of optical, electron and field ion microscope and X-ray diffraction techniques have been used to study the distribution, arrangement and density of dislocations and to determine their properties. To make full use of the information provided by these techniques some understanding of the underlying principles is required. The techniques can be divided into five main groups. (1) Surface methods, in which the point of emergence of a dislocation at the surface of a crystal is revealed. (2) Decoration methods, in which dislocations in bulk specimens transparent to light are decorated with precipitate particles to show up their position. (3) Transmission electron microscopy, in which the dislocations are studied at very high magnification in specimens $0 \cdot 1$ to $4 \cdot 0$ $\mu$m thick. (4) X-ray diffraction, in which local differences in the scattering of X-rays are used to show up the dislocations. (5) Field emission and field ion microscopy, which reveals the position of individual atoms. Except for (5) and isolated examples in (3), these techniques do not reveal directly the arrangement of atoms at the dislocation, but rely on such features as the strain field of the dislocation (Chapter 4) to make them "visible".

## 2.2 Surface Methods

If a crystal containing dislocations is subjected to an environment which removes atoms from the surface the rate of removal of atoms around the point at which a dislocation emerges at the surface may be different from that for the surrounding matrix. The difference in the rate of removal arises from one or more of a number of properties of the dislocation: (1) lattice distortion and strain field of the dislocation; (2) geometry of planes associated with a screw dislocation so that the reverse process to crystal growth produces a surface pit; (3) concentration of impurity atoms at the dislocation which changes the chemical composition of the material near the dislocation. If the rate of removal is more rapid around the dislocation, pits are formed at these sites, Fig. 2.1, and if less rapid small hillocks are formed. Many

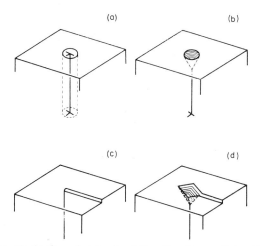

FIG. 2.1. Formation of etch pits at the site where a dislocation meets the surface. (a) Edge dislocation, the cylindrical zone around the dislocation represents the region of the crystal with different physical and chemical properties from the surrounding crystal. (b) Conical shaped pit formed at an edge dislocation due to preferential removal of atoms from the imperfect region. (c) Emergent site of a screw dislocation. (d) Spiral pit formed at a screw dislocation; the pits form by the reverse process to the crystal growth mechanism.

methods are available for the slow, controlled removal of atoms from the surface. The most common and most useful are chemical and electrolytic etching. Other methods include thermal etching, in which the atoms are removed by evaporation when the crystal is heated in a low pressure atmosphere at high temperatures, and cathodic sputtering in which the surface atoms are removed by gas ion bombardment. The last two methods usually reveal only screw dislocations.

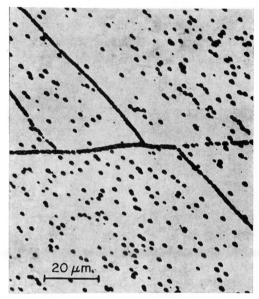

FIG. 2.2. Etch pits produced on the surface of a single crystal of tungsten. (From SCHADLER and Low, unpublished.)

The specimen surface in Fig. 2.2 has been etched and preferential attack has produced black spots identified as pits. It is necessary to establish with some confidence that

(a) dislocations are responsible for the pits, and

(b) all the dislocations meeting the surface have resulted in pits, or alternatively, that all dislocations of the same type have resulted in pits.

A number of methods have been used to confirm this so-called *one-to-one correspondence* between dislocations and etch pits. The first was that due to Vogel and co-workers (1953) which is illustrated in Fig. 2.3. The photograph shows a regularly spaced row of etch pits formed at the boundary between two germanium crystals. Very precise X-ray measurements were made to determine the misorientation between the crystals and is was found that the boundary was a symmetrical pure tilt boundary (section 9.2) which can be described as an array of edge dislocations spaced one above the other as shown in Fig. 2.3(b). Such an array produces a tilt between the grains on opposite sides of the boundary. If $b$ is the strength of the Burgers vector of the edge dislocations and $D$ their distance apart the angle of mis-

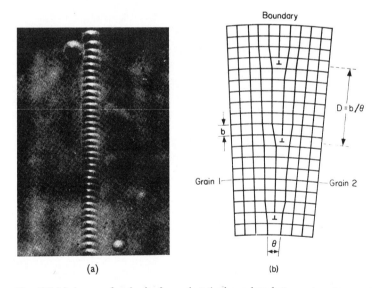

(a)             (b)

FIG. 2.3 (a) A row of etch pits formed at the boundary between two germanium crystals. The etch pits are uniformly spaced. (b) Diagrammatic representation of the arrangement of dislocations in the boundary revealed by the etch pits in (a). This is a symmetrical pure tilt boundary which consists of a vertical array of edge dislocations with parallel Burgers vectors of the same sign. (After VOGEL, PFANN, COREY and THOMAS, *Physical Review* **90**, 489, 1953.)

orientation $\theta$ will be

$$\theta = \frac{b}{D}. \tag{2.1}$$

For the boundary in Fig. 2.3(b) the measured value of $\theta$ was 65 sec of arc, and from equation (2.1) the predicted spacing of dislocations is $1\cdot3 \times 10^{-3}$ mm. This agrees closely with the spacing of the etch pits shown in the photograph confirming that in this example there is a one-to-one correspondence between etch pits and dislocations.

Etch pits have a characteristic shape of conical form which extends to a point at the site of the dislocation. The pits may or may not be perfect crystallographically depending on the electrochemical conditions at the surface of the crystal. The formation and morphology of etch pits is sensitive to the orientation of the crystal surfaces being studied. Thus, for example, Pfann and Vogel (1957) were able to

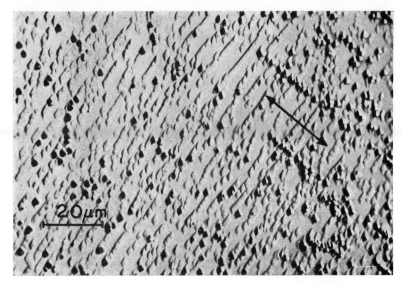

Fig. 2.4. Dark and light etch pits produced at positive and negative edge dislocations in a copper single crystal deformed by slight bending. The arrow indicates the trace of the slip planes. (From LIVINGSTON (1962), *Direct Observations of Imperfections in Crystals*, p. 115, Interscience.)

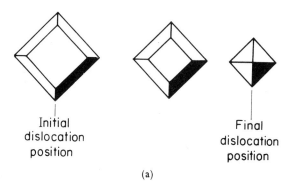

Initial
dislocation
position

Final
dislocation
position

(a)

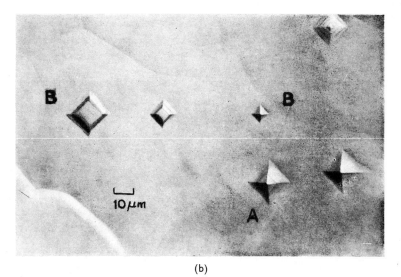

(b)

FIG. 2.5. Etch pits produced on a lithium fluoride crystal. The crystal has been etched three times. The dislocation at *A* has not moved between each etching treatment and a large pyramid shaped pit has formed. The dislocation revealed by the three pits *B* moved between etching treatments to the positions indicated by the pits. Subsequent etching of a pit after the dislocation has moved produces a flat bottom pit. (From GILMAN and JOHNSTON (1957), *Dislocations and Mechanical Properties of Crystals*, p. 116, Wiley.)

etch dislocations in germanium only when the plane of observation was close to (100) or (111). The shape of the etch pit depends also on the character of the dislocation and it is sometimes possible to distinguish between edge and screw dislocations and between positive and negative edge dislocations. A good example of the latter is shown in Fig. 2.4 from work on copper by Livingston (1962).

Although etch pit studies are limited to the surface examination of bulk specimens the technique can be used to study the movement of dislocations as demonstrated by Gilman and Johnston (1957) in lithium fluoride. This is illustrated in Fig. 2.5. The site of a stationary dislocation in a crystal appears as a sharp bottom pit. When a stress is applied to the crystal the dislocation moves; the distance moved depends on the applied stress and the length of time the stress is applied. If the crystal is etched again, the new position of the dislocation is revealed by a new sharp bottom pit. The etchant also attacks the old pit which develops into a flat bottom pit.

In general, surface techniques are limited to crystals with a low dislocation density, less than $10^4$ mm$^{-2}$, because the etch pits have a finite size and are very difficult to resolve when they overlap each other. The distribution of dislocations in three dimensions can be obtained, using this technique, by taking successive sections through the crystal.

## 2.3 Decoration Methods

There are a limited number of crystals which are transparent to light and infra-red radiation. The dislocations in these crystals are not normally visible. However, it is possible to *decorate* the dislocations by inducing precipitation along the line of the dislocation. The effect produced is similar in apperance to a row of beads along a fine thread. The position of the dislocation is revealed by the scattering of the light at the "beads", or precipitates, and can be observed in an optical microscope. In most applications of this method the decoration process involves the heating of the crystals before examination and this restricts the use of the method to the study of "recovered" or high temperature deformation structures. It is not suitable for studying structures formed by low-temperature deformation. The methods used can be classified in terms of the type of crystals examined.

## SILVER HALIDES

The first observation of dislocations using the decoration technique was made by Hedges and Mitchell (1953). It was found that in large transparent crystals of silver bromide and silver chloride, which had been given a suitable thermal treatment, the separation of photolytic silver induced by exposure to light (the print-out process) occurred in regular patterns. These patterns were interpreted as arrays of dislocations on which silver precipitates had formed, thus making them visible.

## ALKALI HALIDES

A technique with a wider range of application, which has been used in studies of defects in NaCl, KCl and KBr, is to dope the crystals with foreign atoms. By suitable heat treatment the precipitation of the foreign atoms can be induced, and they form as small particles or precipitates along the dislocation lines. The size and distribution of the particles can be controlled by the choice of heat treatment. To give a specific example, Amelinckx (1958) decorated the dislocation lines in KCl. The KCl was heavily doped by the addition of 0·75 per cent of AgCl to the melt prior to growth of the crystals. The crystals were annealed in a stream of hydrogen between 650 and 700°C for 3 h. Particles of silver were precipitated on the dislocations in the region of the crystal immediately below the surface. This method has proved of great value in the study of the geometry of dislocation networks or low angle boundaries (Chapter 9). A typical micrograph of an array of dislocations in KCl is shown in Fig. 2.6. The rows of white spots indicate the position of the dislocations.

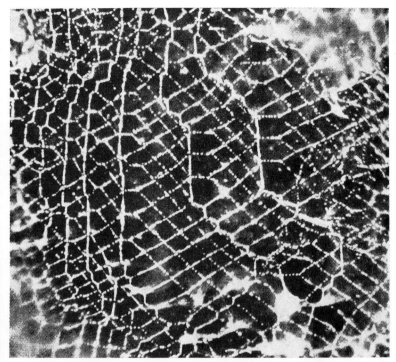

FIG. 2.6. A thin crystal of KCl examined in an optical microscope. Particles of silver have precipitated on the dislocations, which are in the form of a network. Only part of the network is in focus. (From AMELINCKX, *Acta Metall.* **6**, 34, 1958.)

SILICON

The dislocations in silicon can be revealed by the precipitation of copper on the dislocation lines (Dash, 1956). At high temperatures copper diffuses into silicon, but the solubility of copper in silicon decreases rapidly with decreasing temperature below 1200°C and this results in precipitation on cooling to room temperature. The technique usually involves cutting a slice about 1 mm thick out of a single crystal which is then etched. The positions of the dislocations are revealed by the formation of etch pits. The specimens are then

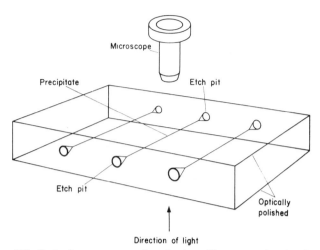

FIG. 2.7. Optical arrangement for viewing silhouettes of etch pits and precipitates associated with the dislocations. (From DASH, J. *Appl. Phys.* **27,** 1193, 1956.)

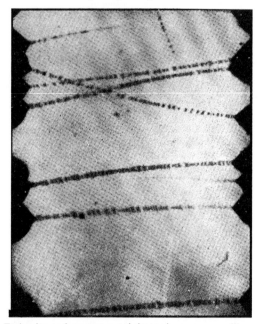

FIG. 2.8. Etch pits and copper precipitates in as-grown silicon. Width of bar is about 1·5 mm, thickness about 1·0 mm. Each row of precipitates marks out a dislocation and extends from an etch pit on one side of the crystal to an etch pit on the other side. (From DASH, *J. Appl. Phys.* **27,** 1193, 1956.)

heated in contact with copper at 900°C in a hydrogen atmosphere and cooled to 20°C. Observation of the precipitates is made with a microscope fitted with an infra-red image tube. Figure 2.7 shows the experimental arrangement and Fig. 2.8 an experimental observation. The rows of fine copper precipitates marking out a dislocation extend from etch pits on one side of the crystal to etch pits on the other side. This observation is a convincing proof of the one-to-one correspondence between dislocations and etch pits for this specimen. The method has been used to study the arrangement of dislocations in as-grown and deformed silicon crystals.

## 2.4 Electron Microscopy

This method has been used to study dislocations, stacking faults, twin and grain boundaries in a wide variety of materials and is potentially applicable to any material which can be produced in very thin sections.

In general the resolution of the electron microscope, say, at best 0·4 nm does not permit the examination of the atomic arrangement around the dislocation and the observation of dislocations is only possible because of the scattering of electrons in the strained region around the dislocation. The technique based on this approach is called *transmission electron microscopy*. There are two outstanding, but very specialised, exceptions to this generalisation and these are described before the more universal method.

MOIRÉ FRINGES

An effect, well known in optics, was used by Pashley, Menter and Bassett to produce an effective magnification of the spacing between atom planes. In metals this spacing is 0·2 nm and therefore less than the resolution of the electron microscope. The formation of Moiré fringes is illustrated in Fig. 2.9. When two parallel sets of lines, with spacing $d_1$ and $d_2$, are superimposed an enlarged pattern of parallel fringes is produced with a spacing $(d_1 d_2)/(d_2 - d_1)$ giving a Moiré magnification $d_1/(d_2 - d_1)$. When one of the set of lines contains an arrangement similar to a section through a lattice normal to an edge dislocation, there is again a magnification effect. In an analogous way dislocations can be revealed by superimposing two

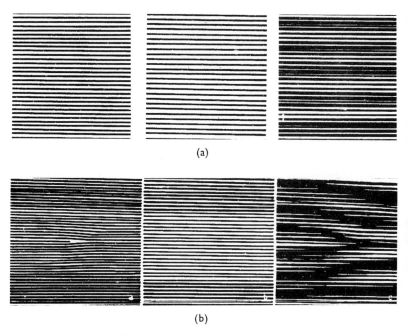

(a)

(b)

FIG. 2.9. (a) Optical analogue to illustrate the formation of magnified images, Moiré fringes, by superimposing parallel lines with differing spacings. (b) Optical analogue to illustrate the formation of a dislocation in the Moiré pattern. (After AMELINCKX and DEKEYSER, *Solid State Physics*, **8**, 327, 1959).

crystals with the same crystal structure but different lattice parameters. In the simplest example the two lattices must be closely parallel and this is achieved by depositing one film upon another epitaxially. The example shown in Fig. 2.10 was obtained by depositing a layer of palladium ($d_{1(02\bar{2})} = 0\cdot137$ nm) on to a (111) gold film ($d_{2(02\bar{2})} = 0\cdot144$ nm) giving a Moiré magnification of $\sim 20$. The dislocation

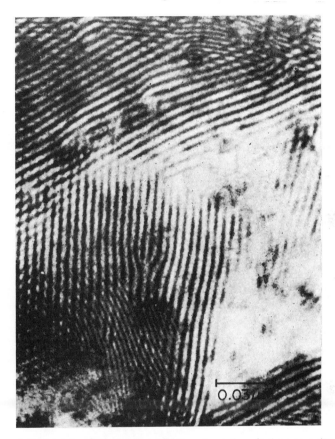

FIG. 2.10. Moiré pattern from a palladium layer deposited on to a (111) gold film. "Dislocations" in the pattern correspond to dislocations in the metal film. In this example, the prominent dislocation contains two extra half planes. (From BASSETT, MENTER and PASHLEY, *Proc. Roy. Soc.* A, **246**, 345, 1958.)

image in the photograph has two terminating half-planes due to the particular type of dislocation which forms in face-centred cubic metals (see section 5.3). This method has a very limited application mainly because of the stringent requirements for producing the contrast from the specimen and the difficulty of specimen preparation.

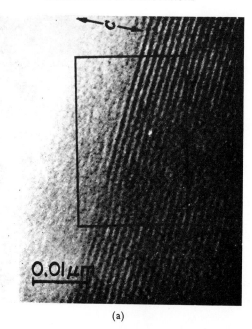

(a)

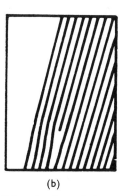

(b)

FIG. 2.11. (a) Single edge dislocation in a platinum phthalocyanine crystal. (b) Guide to marked area in (a) to show the position of the edge dislocation. (From MENTER, *Proc. Roy. Soc.* A, **236,** 119, 1956.)

MOLECULAR CRYSTALS

When crystals with lattice spacings greater than the microscope resolution are studied it is possible, using an appropriate electron optical arrangement, to observe dislocations directly. Such observations have been made by Menter (1956) on thin crystals of copper and platinum phthalocyanine, in which the spacing of atom planes is ~1·2 nm. A well-known example is shown in Fig. 2.11 along with a line diagram to indicate the position of the dislocation.

GENERAL APPLICATION—TRANSMISSION ELECTRON MICROSCOPY

In X-ray diffraction, X-rays incident on a crystal are diffracted by parallel sets of atom planes in a similar way the reflection of light by a plane mirror. The position of the diffracted beams satisfy the *Bragg reflection* conditions. In a similar way an electron beam is scattered by a crystal. Dislocations and stacking faults can be revealed by a technique which examines the interference between transmitted and diffracted beams resulting from a beam of electrons incident on a very thin foil of a crystal, usually between 100 and 500 nm thick. The method of forming images of the diffracted beams is illustrated in Fig. 2.12. A parallel beam of electrons, usually accelerated by a potential of 100 kV, is transmitted through a thin foil *AB* and is diffracted in a number of directions by the crystal. The diffracted beams are brought to a focus in the back focal plane *CD* of the objective lens thus forming a *diffraction pattern* which can be suitably magnified and studied if subsequent lenses in the microscope are arranged to focus on the plane *CD*. The diffraction pattern consists of an approximately two-dimensional array of spots, each spot corresponding to a particular set of reflecting planes. The orientation of the foil can be determined from this pattern.

Each spot in the diffraction pattern is produced by the diffraction of the incident beam from a relatively large area of the specimen (approximately $10^4$ atom spacings in diameter). Figure 2.12 shows that an image of the lower surface of the specimen is formed by the objective lens in the plane *EF*. This image can be magnified by other lenses in the instrument. If all the diffracted beams contribute to this image the quality of the image is poor mainly because of lens aberra-

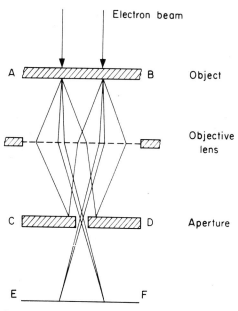

FIG. 2.12. Diagram illustrating the formation of images in the electron microscope. An incident beam of electrons is diffracted by the specimen and the diffracted beams are stopped by the objective aperture. Contrast in the image produced at *EF* by the main transmitted beam arises through local variations in the intensities of the diffracted beams. (From WHELAN, *J. Inst. Metals*, **87**, 392, 1958–9.)

tion. However, the image resulting from a single beam can be obtained by inserting an objective aperture. Two main possibilities exist. Firstly, the aperture is centred on the main transmitted beam producing a so-called *bright field image*, and secondly, the aperture is centred over a diffracted beam producing a *dark field image*. Most work is done using bright field illumination, but there are important applications for dark field illumination.

For a perfectly flat specimen containing no defects, a completely homogeneous image is expected when the objective aperture is centred over the main transmitted beam. Changes in the brightness of the image are produced by any effect which changes the path of a diffracted beam so that it enters the objective aperture and interferes with the transmitted beam. A good demonstration of this is provided by the buckling of the very thin foils used in these studies. The orientation of the specimen relative to the electron beam varies slightly in different parts of the specimen and therefore the local reflection conditions governed by the Bragg law vary also. The interference between transmitted and diffracted beams produces variations in the intensity of the bright field image called *extinction contours* which appear as dark bands across the image indicating that a set of planes near the bands are in a strongly diffracting orientation. When bending of the foil occurs in the microscope, during observation of the foil, the extinction contours appear to move across the specimen.

This simplified approach can be used to account for the contrast produced by dislocations. In Fig. 1.15(b) it is shown that the planes near the dislocation are bent slightly and therefore the diffraction conditions at the dislocation will be different than in the surrounding perfect crystal. Considering bright field illumination, if the planes are bent locally into a diffracting position so that interference occurs the transmitted intensity will be smaller and the dislocation will appear as a dark line, see Fig. 2.13. The width of the dark line is usually about 10 nm and is much wider than the actual dislocation. It must be emphasised that the observation of the dislocation in this way arises from a diffraction effect, and depending on the precise diffraction conditions the dislocation will produce a number of different images such as, (1) single dark line on one side of the dislocation, (2) two dark lines, (3) dotted line, (4) wavy line, (5) no change in contrast so that the dilocation is not visible. The last contrast effect mentioned is widely used to determine the Burgers vectors of dislocations. It occurs when the principal diffracting planes producing the image contrast are not tilted by the presence of the dislocation,

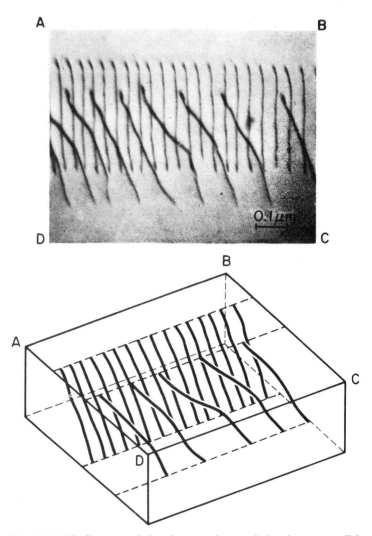

FIG. 2.13. Thin film transmission electron micrograph showing two parallel rows of dislocations. Each dark line is produced by a dislocation. The dislocations extend from top to bottom of the foil which is about 200 nm thick. The line diagram illustrates the distribution of the dislocations in the foil and demonstrates that the photograph above represents a projected image of a three-dimensional array of dislocations.

i.e. those planes which contain the Burgers vector **b**, since, to a first approximation these planes remain flat when a dislocation is introduced. The condition for this to occur is $\mathbf{g} \cdot \mathbf{b} = 0$ where **g** is a vector normal to the reflecting planes. An example of the use of this technique is illustrated in Fig. 2.14. The different contrast patterns in the three photographs of the *same* field of view are due to the use of three different sets of reflecting planes in the crystal. The network contains four sets of dislocations with different Burgers vectors. By changing the imaging reflection it is possible to bring different sets of dislocations into contrast.

Stacking faults also produce a characteristic diffraction image. A stacking fault is produced by the displacement of one part of a crystal by a constant vector **R** relative to the other half (section 1.4). The effect of a stacking fault (with **R** in the plane of the fault) on the reflecting planes is shown in Fig. 2.15. When the fault vector lies in the plane of the fault which is parallel to the reflecting planes there is no change in contrast (Fig. 2.15a). This is an example of the $\mathbf{g} \cdot \mathbf{b} = 0$ condition mentioned above, where $\mathbf{R} = \mathbf{b}$. However, when **R** does not lie in the reflecting planes $\mathbf{g} \cdot \mathbf{R} \neq 0$, as in Fig. 2.15(b). The planes are out of register at the fault, and interference between electrons reflected from planes above and below the fault gives rise to a fringe pattern in the image. The fringes run parallel to the intersection of the foil surfaces with the plane containing the stacking fault, Fig. 2.16. Similar fringe patterns are produced at twin boundaries and grain boundaries inclined at an angle to the plane of the foil.

The study of defects by this technique is applicable to all materials which can be prepared in sufficiently thin sections. The limiting factor determining the thickness of the foil is the absorption of electrons. In general, metals with a high atomic number absorb electrons more effectively than those with low atomic numbers and must be prepared in thinner sections. The method of preparing thin sections or foils is dictated by the nature of the material and the properties being studied. If the conditions of the experiment allow, the simplest method of preparing metal foils is (a) roll the metal into a sheet about 10 $\mu$m thick, (b) apply the thermal and mechanical

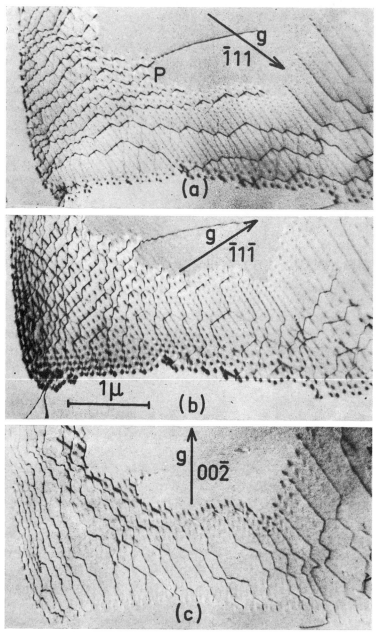

FIG. 2.14. Illustration of the use of the $\mathbf{g} \cdot \mathbf{b} = 0$ method to determine the Burgers vector of dislocations. (From LINDROOS, *Phil. Mag.* **24,** 709, 1971).

treatment to be investigated (c) thin to 100–500 nm by electropolishing, chemical polishing or ion beam etching. It is often difficult to produce homogeneous thinning in the last stage, and various techniques have been developed to improve this. It may be necessary to examine thin sections of bulk materials of both metals and non-metals already in the final thermal and mechanical condition. To do this a slice is cut out, either by very careful machining or by spark erosion and this is then thinned by chemical polishing electrolytic polishing

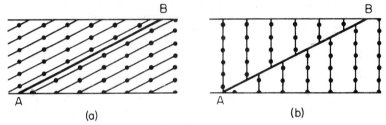

FIG. 2.15. Displacements of the reflecting planes at a stacking fault *AB*. In (a) **g·R** = 0 and no contrast occurs. In (b) **g·R** ≠ 0 and interference between waves from above and below the fault gives a fringe pattern. (From HOWIE, *Metallurgical Reviews*, **6**, 467, 1961).

or ion beam etching. It is important to avoid introducing deformation in the metal during preparation because this will affect the density and distribution of the defects being studied. Many other more specialised techniques have been used, for example, very thin flakes of single crystals of zinc can be prepared by deposition from the vapour and sections of graphite and other layer type structures can be obtained merely by scraping the surface of the bulk material.

Using transmission electron microscopy three-dimensional arrangements of dislocations can be observed in crystals about 200 nm thick. The interaction between dislocations can be observed directly. Movement of the dislocations can be induced by straining the thin sections in the microscope using a miniature tensile stage (specimens are approximately 2·5 mm long). It is possible to obtain quantitative measurements of the density of dislocations providing the thickness of the foil can be measured. There are certain limitations which

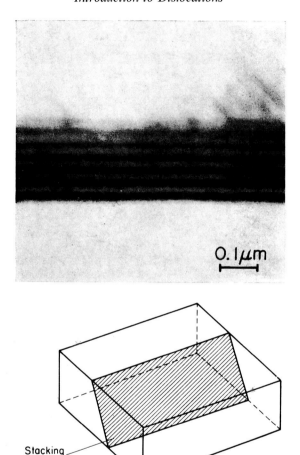

FIG. 2.16. Thin film transmission electron micrograph showing the fringe pattern typical of stacking faults, twin boundaries and grain boundaries which lie at an angle to the plane of the foil.

must be borne in mind when using the method, principally, that the arrangement of dislocations and their mutal interaction may be modified in very thin sections compared with bulk material. This difficulty, amongst others, has led to the development of *high voltage*

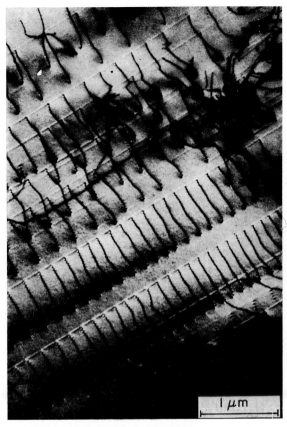

Fig. 2.17. Arrays of dislocations in a stainless steel specimen about 2µm thick photographed using an electron microscope operating at 1 MV. (From DUPOUY and PERRIER, *J. de Microscopie* **1**, 167, 1962.)

*electron microscopy* with accelerating voltages of 1 MV, and in one case up to 3 MV. Using high accelerating voltages it is possible to examine some metal specimens up to 2 to 4 µm thick. An early example from the first 1 MV electron microscope is shown in Fig. 2.17.

Another important development in electron microscopy has been the use of the *weak beam technique*. This involves obtaining an image

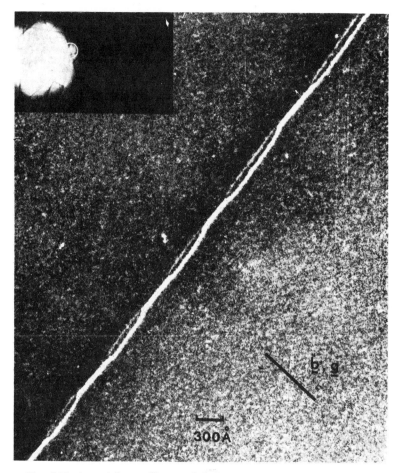

FIG. 2.18. A weak-beam 22U dark-field image oı a dislocation in an annealed silicon specimen showing constricted segments. The inset shows the diffracting conditions used to form the image. (From RAY and COCKAYNE, *Proc. Roy. Soc.* **A 325,** 543, 1971)

of the dislocation strain field by selecting a reflecting condition such that reflections only occur from planes close to the centre of the dislocation which are bent locally by the presence of the dislocation. The advantage of this technique is that the width of the observed dislocation image is reduced from about 10 nm to 1 to 2 nm so that it is possible to resolve dislocations which are very closely spaced. An example is shown in Fig. 2.18.

## 2.5 X-ray Diffraction Topography

Direct observation of dislocations with X-rays is achieved by a method somewhat similar to electron diffraction, but with a greatly reduced resolution. Consequently, it is applicable only to the study of crystals with low dislocation densities $\sim 10^4$ mm$^{-2}$, but has the advantage that the penetration of X-rays is greater than electrons so that much thicker specimens can be used. The specimen, usually a large single crystal is oriented with respect to the X-ray beam so that a set of lattice planes is set at the Bragg angle for strong reflection. The reflected beam is examined photographically. As in electron diffraction, any local bending of the lattice associated with a dislocation results in a change in the reflection conditions and the X-rays are scattered differently in this region. The difference in the intensity of the diffracted X-rays can be recorded photographically. A photograph of dislocations in a silicon crystal revealed by X-ray diffraction topography is show in Fig. 2.19.

## 2.6 Field Ion Microscopy

The maximum resolution of the electron microscope does not allow the examination of the positions of individual atoms and, in particular, point defects cannot be detected unless they form in clusters. This limitation has been overcome by the development of the field ion microscope which has a resolution of 0·2 to 0·3 nm. The specimen is a fine wire which is electro-polished at one end to a sharp hemispherical tip 100–300 atoms in radius. A map of the atom positions at this tip can be obtained. The specimen tip is positively charged to 5–15 kV and is surrounded by a high vacuum with a trace of helium or neon gas. The atoms at the surface are ionised by the high positive charge and when a helium atom approaches it gives

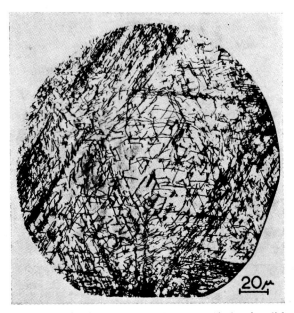

FIG. 2.19. X-ray diffraction topograph (micrograph) showing dislocations
in a single crystal of silicon. No magnification occurs in recording the
topograph, but by using very fine grain sized photographic emulsions
subsequent magnification up to about ×500 is possible. (From JENKINSON
and LANG (1962), *Direct Observation of Imperfections in Crystals*, p. 471,
Interscience.)

up an electron to the metal and becomes positively charged. The
helium atom then accelerates down the lines of force radiating from
the metal ion and produces an image of the ion on a screen which
can be photographed. Since the ions travel approximately perpendicular to the local tip surface there is a *geometrical* magnification of
about $d/r$, where $r$ is the tip radius and $d$ is the distance from the
specimen to the fluorescent screen. Each atom appears as a bright
spot.

Only a certain number of the atoms at the tip (approximately 1 in
5) are ionised and produce an image, but characteristic patterns
are formed from which it is possible to deduce the positions of all
the other atoms. When an atom is missing, i.e. a vacancy, one of

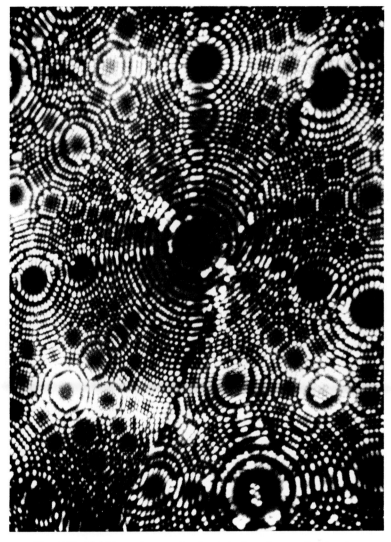

FIG. 2.20. Field ion micrograph of a grain boundary at the tip of a tungsten needle. Each bright spot represents a tungsten atom. (From *Scientific American*, Sept. 1967.)

the white spots is missing. A particularly striking demonstration of the potentialities of the method has been made by Brandon and Wald who photographed the tip of a tungsten wire before and after irradiation with α-particles. After irradiation many of the bright spots were missing, indicating that the atoms had been knocked out of their atomic sites (i.e. vacancies had been formed) by the α-particles. An example of a field ion micrograph is shown in Fig. 2.20. The structure of the grain boundary closely resembles that observed using the bubble raft, Fig. 1.20.

Field ion microscopy is restricted to the examination of very small areas and only atomic arrangements at the free surface can be revealed. However, for any application which requires exact information of the positions of individual atoms, this technique is invaluable.

## Further Reading

AMELINCKX, S. (1964) "The direct observation of dislocations", *Solid State Physics* Supplement 6.

BRANDON, D. G. (1966) *Modern Techniques in Metallography*, Butterworths.

BRANDON, D. G. (1971) *Cambridge Conference on Electron Microscopy and Analysis* Institute of Physics, London.

GEVERS, R., AMELINCKX, S., REMAUT, G. and VAN LANDUYT, I. (Eds.) (1970) *Modern Diffraction and Imaging Techniques in Materials Science*, North Holland Press.

HIRSCH, P. B., HOWIE, A., NICHOLSON, R. B. and PASHLEY, D. W. (1965) *Electron Microscopy of Thin Crystals*, Butterworth.

JOHNSTON, W. G. (1962) "Dislocation etch pits in non-metallic crystals", *Progress in Ceramic Science*, Vol. 2, Pergamon Press.

MÜLLER, E. W. and TSONG, T. T. (1969) *Field Ion Microscopy*, Elsevier.

NEWKIRK, J. B. and WERNICK, J. H. (Eds.) (1962) *Direct Observations of Imperfections in Crystals*, Interscience.

PASHLEY, D. W. (1965) "The direct observation of imperfections in crystals", *Reports on Prog. in Phys.* **28**, 291.

THOMAS, G. (1962) *Transmission Electron Microscopy of Metals*, Wiley.

THOMAS, G. FULRATH, R. M. and FISHER, R. M. (Eds.) (1972) *Electron Microscopy and Structure of Materials*, University of California Press.

CHAPTER 3

# Movement of Dislocations

## 3.1 Concept of Slip

There are two basic types of dislocation movement, *glide* or *conservative motion* in which the dislocation moves in the surface which contains both its line and Burgers vector, and *climb* or *non-conservative motion* in which the dislocation moves out of the glide surface normal to the Burgers vector. The subject is approached from a consideration of the concept of *slip* which is the most common manifestation of glide. This approach provides also a valuable understanding of the structure of the dislocation.

Plastic deformation in a crystal occurs by the sliding or successive displacement of one plane of atoms over another on so-called *slip planes*. Discrete blocks of crystal between two slip planes remain undistorted as illustrated in Fig. 3.1. Further deformation occurs either by more movement on existing slip planes or by the formation of new slip planes. The slip plane is normally the plane with the highest density of atoms and the direction of slip is the direction in the slip plane in which the atoms are most closely spaced. Thus, in close-packed hexagonal crystals, slip often occurs on the (0001) basal plane in directions of the type $\langle \bar{1}2\bar{1}0 \rangle$ and in face-centred cubic metals on $\{111\}$ planes in $\langle 110 \rangle$ directions. In body-centred cubic crystals the slip direction is the $\langle 111 \rangle$ close-packed direction, but the slip plane is not well defined on a macroscopic scale. Microscopic evidence suggests that slip occurs on $\{112\}$ and $\{110\}$ planes and that

{110} slip is preferred at low temperatures. A slip plane and a slip direction in the plane constitute a *slip system*. Face-centred cubic crystals have four {111} planes and three ⟨110⟩ directions, and therefore have twelve {111} ⟨110⟩ slip systems. Slip results in the formation of steps on the surface of the crystal. These are readily detected

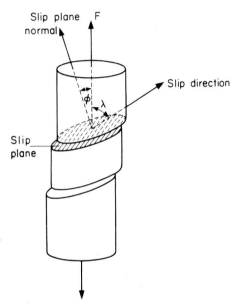

FIG. 3.1. Illustration of the geometry of slip in crystalline materials.

if the surface is carefully polished before plastic deformation. Figure 3.2 is an example of slip in a 3·25 per cent silicon iron crystal; the line diagram illustrates the appearance of a section through the crystal normal to the surface.

A characteristic shear stress is required for slip. Consider the crystal illustrated in Fig. 3.1 which is being deformed in tension by an applied force $F$ along the axis of the cylindrical crystal. If the cross-sectional area is $A$ the tensile stress parallel to $F$ is $\sigma = F/A$. The force has a component $F \cos \lambda$ in the slip direction, where $\lambda$ is the angle between $F$ and the slip direction. This force acts over the slip surface which has an area $A/\cos \phi$, where $\phi$ is the angle between $F$ and the normal to the slip plane. Thus the shear stress $\tau$, resolved on the slip plane in the slip direction, is

$$\tau = \frac{F}{A} \cos \phi \cos \lambda. \tag{3.1}$$

If $F_c$ is the tensile force required to start slip, the corresponding value of the shear stress $\tau_c$ is called the *critical resolved shear stress for slip*. It has been found in some metal crystals which deform on a single slip system that $\tau_c$ is independent of the orientation of the crystal.

### 3.2 Dislocations and Slip

In Chapter 1 it was shown that the theoretical shear stress for slip was many times greater than the experimentally observed stress, i.e. $\tau_c$. The low value can be accounted for by the movement of dislocations. Consider the edge dislocation represented in Fig. 1.15. This could be formed in a different way to that described in Chapter 1, as follows: cut a slot along *AEFD* in the crystal shown in Fig. 3.3 and displace the top half of the crystal above *AEFD* one lattice spacing over the bottom half in the direction $\overrightarrow{AB}$. An extra half plane *EFGH* and a dislocation line *FE* are formed, although it is emphasised that dislocations are not formed in this way in practice. The dislocation can be defined as the *boundary between the slipped and unslipped parts of the crystal*. Apart from the region around the dislocations the atoms across *AEFD* are in perfect register. Only a relatively small applied stress is required to move the dislocation along the plane *ABCD* in the way demonstrated in Fig. 3.4. This can be understood from the following argument. In the perfect lattice all the atoms above and below the slip plane are in minimum energy positions and when the atoms are displaced the same force acts on all the atoms, opposing the movement. When there is a dislocation in the lattice the atoms well away from the dislocation are still in the minimum energy position but at the dislocation they are not. The atoms around the dislocation are symmetrically placed on opposite sides of the extra half

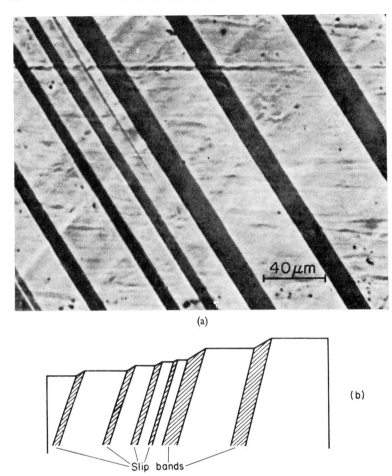

(a)

(b)

FIG. 3.2. (a) Straight slip bands on a single crystal of 3·25 per cent silicon iron. (From HULL, *Proc. Roy. Soc.* A, **274**, 5, 1963.) (b) Sketch of a section across the slip bands normal to surface shown in (a). Each band is made up of a large number of slip steps on closely spaced parallel slip planes.

plane and provide equal and opposite forces on the atoms at the dislocation. In this over-simplified description there is no net force on the dislocation and the stress required to move the dislocation is zero. In practice, certain symmetry conditions give rise to a lattice resistance to the movement of a dislocation which is referred to as the *Peierls–Nabarro force* (see Chapter 10) but this is much smaller than the theoretical shear stress of a perfect lattice.

The movement of the dislocation, from one position to the next (Fig. 3.4), involves only a small rearrangement of the atomic bonds near the dislocation. The movement of one dislocation across the

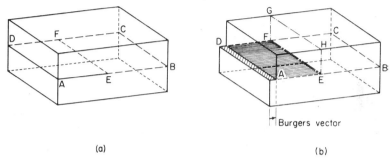

FIG. 3.3. Formation of a pure edge dislocation *FE*.

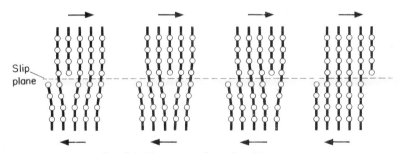

FIG. 3.4. Movement of an edge dislocation.

slip plane to the surface of the crystal produces a slip step equal to the Burgers vector of the dislocation. The slip direction is necessarily always parallel to the Burgers vector of the dislocation responsible for slip. The plastic strain resulting from dislocation movement can be determined in the following way: if an element of dislocation, Burgers vector **b**, sweeps out an area $A$ of a slip plane total area

$A_s$, the two halves of the crystal will be displaced $(A/A_s)b$, relative to each other, and the increment of plastic strain will be $(A/A_s)b/V$ where $V$ is the volume of the crystal, (see section 10.7).

### 3.3 The Slip Plane

In Fig. 3.3 the edge dislocation has moved in the plane *ABCD* which is the *slip plane*. This is uniquely defined by the position of the dislocation line and the Burgers vector of the dislocation. The

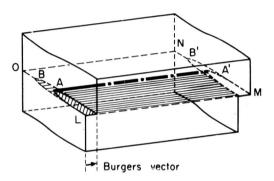

Fɪɢ. 3.5. Formation and movement of a pure screw dislocation *AA'* to *BB'* by slip.

movement of an edge dislocation is limited, therefore, to a specific plane. The movement of a screw dislocation, for example from *AA'* to *BB'* in Fig. 3.5, can also be envisaged to take place in a slip plane, i.e. *LMNO*, and a slip step is formed. However, the line of the screw dislocation and the Burgers vector do not define a plane and the movement of the dislocation is not restricted to a specific plane. It will be noted that the displacement of atoms and hence the slip step associated with the movement of a screw dislocation is parallel to the dislocation line. This can be demonstrated further by considering a plan view of the atoms above and below a slip plane containing a screw dislocation, Fig. 3.6. Movement of the screw dislocation produces a displacement *b* parallel to the dislocation line.

In the two examples illustrated in Figs. 3.3 and 3.5, it has been assumed that the moving dislocations remained straight. However, dislocations are generally bent and irregular, particularly after plastic deformation. A more general shape of a dislocation is shown in Fig. 3.7. The boundary separating the slipped and unslipped regions of the crystal is curved, i.e. the dislocation is curved, but the Burgers

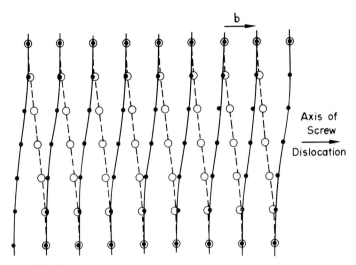

Fɪɢ. 3.6. Arrangement of atoms around a screw dislocations.

vector is the same all along its length. It follows that at point *C* the dislocation line is *normal* to the vector and is therefore *pure edge* and at *A* is *parallel* to the vector and is *pure screw*. The remainder of the dislocation has a *mixed edge and screw* character. The Burgers vector **b** of a mixed dislocation, *xy* in Fig. 3.7(b), can be resolved into two components by regarding the dislocation as two coincident dislocations; a pure edge with vector $\mathbf{b}_1$ at right angles to *xy*, and a pure screw with vector $\mathbf{b}_2$ parallel to *xy*.

$$\mathbf{b}_1 + \mathbf{b}_2 = \mathbf{b} \tag{3.2}$$

It is emphasised that this has no physical significance.

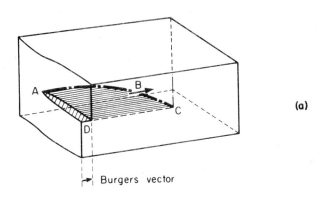

(a)

Burgers vector

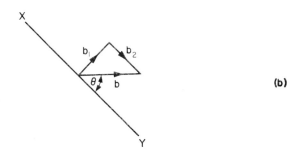

(b)

Fig. 3.7. Mixed dislocations. (a) The curved dislocation *ABC* is pure edge at *C* and pure screw at *A*. (b) Burgers vector **b** of dislocation *XY* is resolved into a pure edge component **b₁** and a pure screw component **b₂**.

### 3.4 Cross Slip

In general, screw dislocations tend to move in certain crystallographic planes (see, for example, dissociation of unit dislocations, section 5.3). Thus, in face-centred cubic metals the screw dislocations move in {111} type planes, but can switch from one {111} type plane to another. This process, known as *cross slip*, is illustrated in Fig. 3.8. In Fig. 3.8(a) a small loop of dislocation line, Burgers vector $\mathbf{b} = \frac{1}{2}$ [$\bar{1}01$], is expanding in the (111) plane under the action of a small applied shear stress. At $w$ and $y$ the dislocation is a pure positive and a pure negative edge dislocation respectively, and at $x$ and $z$ the dislocation is a right-handed and a left-handed screw dislocation respectively. Let us suppose that as the loop expands the local stress field which is producing dislocation motion changes so that

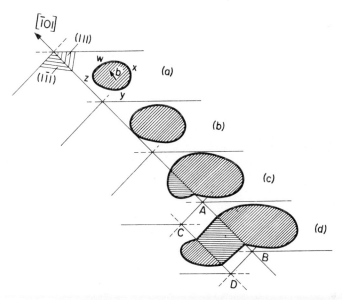

FIG. 3.8. Cross slip in a face-centred cubic crystal. The [$\bar{1}01$] direction is common to (111) and (1$\bar{1}$1) close-packed planes. A screw dislocation at $z$ is free to glide in either of these planes. Cross slip produces a non-planar slip surface. Double cross slip is shown in (d).

motion is preferred on (1$\bar{1}$1) instead of (111). This is illustrated in Fig. 3.8 (b) and (c). The dislocation at $z$ is pure screw and is free to move in both (1$\bar{1}$1) and (111) planes so that further expansion of the loop occurs in the (1$\bar{1}$1) plane. *Double cross slip* is illustrated in Fig. 3.8(d). An example of cross slip is shown in Fig. 3.9. The cross slip of moving dislocations is readily seen by transmission electron microscopy because a moving dislocation leaves a track which slowly

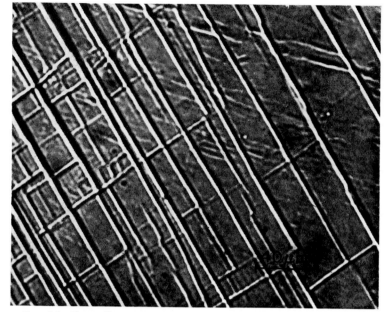

FIG. 3.9. Cross slip on the polished surface of a single crystal of 3·25 per cent silicon iron.

fades. In body-centred cubic metals the slip plane is less well defined and the screw dislocation often wanders from one plane to another producing wavy slip lines on prepolished surfaces.

## 3.5 Velocity of Dislocations

Dislocations move by glide at velocities which depend on the applied shear stress, purity of crystal, temperature and type of dislocation. A direct method of measuring dislocation velocity was developed by Johnston and Gilman using etch pits to reveal the position of dislocations at different stages of deformation as illustrated in Fig. 2.5. A crystal containing freshly introduced dislocations, usually produced by lightly deforming the surface, is subjected to a constant stress pulse for a given time. From the positions of the dislocations before and after the stress pulse, the distance each dislocation has moved, and hence the average dislocation velocity, can be determined. By repeating the experiment for different times and stress levels the velocity can be determined as a function of stress as shown in Fig. 3.10a for lithium fluoride. The dislocation velocity was measured over twelve orders of magnitude and was a very sensitive function of the resolved shear stress. In the range of velocities between $10^{-7}$ and $10^{-1}$ cm sec$^{-1}$ the logarithm of the velocity varies

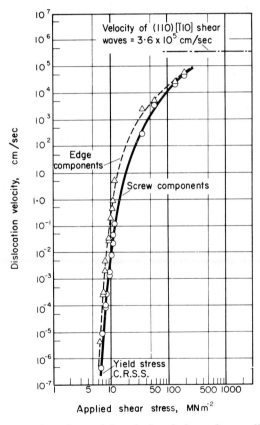

FIG. 3.10a Stress dependence of the velocity of edge and screw dislocations in lithium fluoride. (From JOHNSTON and GILMAN, *J. Appl. Phys.* **30**, 129, 1959.)

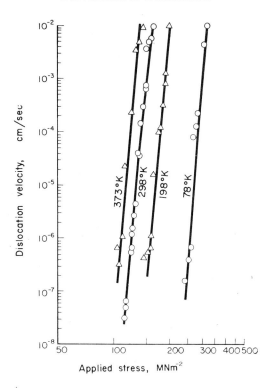

FIG. 3.10b Stress dependence of the velocity of edge dislocations in 3·25 per cent silicon iron at four temperatures. (After STEIN and LOW, *J. Appl. Phys.* **31**, 362, 1960.)

linearly with the logarithm of the applied stress, thus

$$v \propto \left( \frac{\tau}{\tau_0} \right)^n \qquad (3.3a)$$

Where $v$ is velocity, $\tau$ is the applied shear stress resolved in the slip plane, $\tau_0$ is the shear stress for $v = 1$ cm sec$^{-1}$, $n$ is a constant and was found experimentally to be $\sim 25$ for lithium fluoride. It must be emphasised that equation (3.3a) is purely empirical and implies no physical interpretation of the mechanism of dislocation motion.

It is probably more realistic to use an expression of the form

$$v = v_0 \exp\left(-\frac{A}{\tau}\right) \tag{3.3b}$$

where $v_0$ and $A$ are constants which depend on the material. For velocities greater than 10 cm sec$^{-1}$ the velocity does not increase as rapidly with increasing stress and it tends to an upper limit close to the velocity of shear wave propagation in this material. The velocity of edge and screw components was measured independently and in the low velocity range edge dislocations moved 50 times faster than screw dislocations. There is a critical stress, which represents the onset of plastic deformation, required to start the dislocations moving. The effect of temperature on dislocation velocity is illustrated in Fig. 3.10b for results obtained by Stein and Low who studied 3·25 per cent silicon iron by the same method. The dislocation velocities were only measured below 10$^{-2}$ cm sec$^{-1}$ and therefore the curves do not show the bending over found in lithium fluoride. The curves

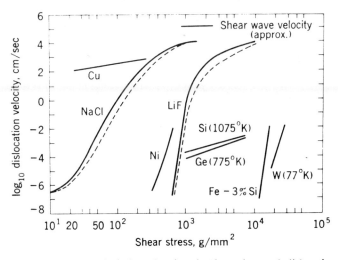

FIG. 3.11. Some typical data showing the dependence of dislocation velocities on applied stress. (After GILMAN, *Micromechanics of flow in Solids*, McGraw-Hill).

are of the same form as equation (3.3a). At 293 K, $n \sim 35$, and at 78 K, $n \sim 44$. $\tau_0$ increased with decreasing temperature.

These experiments are now being repeated using high voltage electron microscopy (see, for example, T. Imura in *Electron microscopy and strength of materials*). It is possible to strain the crystal under controlled conditions and follow the motion of dislocations directly. The results indicate the same kind of stress dependence revealed using the pulse technique and etch pit studies, but the velocities of both edge and screw dislocations are found to be much higher. This means that the average velocity of dislocations over long distances such as those involved in etch pit work is much smaller by a factor of $10^2$ than the velocity over short distances. The stress dependence of dislocation velocity varies significantly from one material to another as illustrated in Fig. 3.11.

### 3.6 Climb

At low temperatures where diffusion is difficult, and in the absence of a non-equilibrium concentration of point defects, the movement of dislocations is restricted almost entirely to glide. However, at higher temperatures an edge dislocation can move out of its slip plane by a process called *climb*. Consider the diagram of an edge dislocation in Fig. 3.12. If the row of atoms $A$ normal to the plane of the diagram is removed, the dislocation line moves up one atom spacing out of its original slip plane; this is called *positive climb*. Similarly, if a row of atoms is introduced below the extra half plane the dislocation line moves down one atom spacing, *negative climb*. Positive climb can occur by either diffusion of vacancies to $A$ or the formation of an interstitial atom at $A$ and its diffusion away. Negative climb can occur either by an interstitial atom diffusing to $A$ or the formation of a vacancy at $A$ and its diffusion away. All these processes require mass transport by diffusion and therefore climb requires thermal activation. The most common climb processes involve the diffusion of vacancies either towards or away from the dislocation.

It has been assumed above that a complete row of atoms is re-

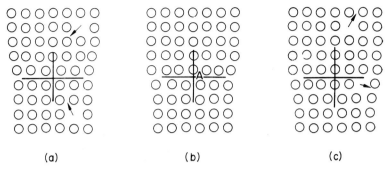

(a)                    (b)                    (c)

FIG. 3.12. Positive and negative climb of an edge dislocation. In (b) the dislocation is centred on the row of atoms *A* normal to the plane of the diagram. If the vacancies in the lattice diffuse to the dislocation at *A* the dislocation will climb in a positive sense as in (a). If vacancies are generated at the dislocation line and then diffuse away the dislocation will climb in the negative sense as in (c).

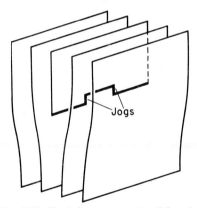

FIG. 3.13. Single jogs on an edge dislocation.

moved simultaneously, whereas in practice individual vacancies or small clusters of vacancies diffuse to the dislocation. The effect of this is illustrated in Fig. 3.13 which shows climb of a short section of a dislocation line resulting in the formation of two steps called *jogs*. Both positive and negative climb proceeds by the nucleation and motion of jogs. Conversely, jogs are *sources* and *sinks* for vacancies.

The jogs described have a height of one lattice spacing and have a characteristic energy $U_j \approx 0.16$ aJ (1 eV) (see section 7.1). There will be a thermodynamic equilibrium number of jogs per unit length of a dislocation

$$n_j = n_0 \exp\left(-\frac{U_j}{kT}\right) \tag{3.4}$$

where $n_0$ is the number of atom sites per unit length of dislocation. If $U_v$ is the energy of formation of a vacancy and $U_m$ is the energy

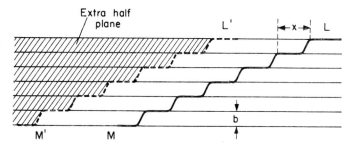

FIG. 3.14. Climb of an edge dislocation by the movement of jogs. The edge dislocation *LM* contains jogs distance *x* apart. Diffusion of vacancies to the jogs moves the dislocation to *L'M'*.

of movement of a vacancy, the activation energy of climb in thermal equilibrium will be

$$U_c = U_j + U_v + U_m = U_j + U_d \tag{3.5}$$

where $U_d$ is the activation energy for self-diffusion. If the dislocations are heavily jogged by prior plastic deformation (see Chapter 7) or a ready site for jog formation is available which does not involve thermal nucleation, climb will be determined only by the energy for self diffusion.

The rate of climb depends on many factors, some of which can be understood by referring to Fig. 3.14. The edge dislocation *LM* lies at an angle to the glide plane and has a Burgers vector normal to the plane of the diagram. The distance between jogs on *LM* is *x*. Positive climb of the dislocation will move the dislocation line up

to $L'M'$ without removing the jogs. The unit process is the movement of a jog along the dislocation line and the velocity of the jog
determines the rate of climb. The velocity of a jog depends on two
principal factors. Firstly, the force due to an applied stress which
tends to make the jog emit vacancies and move the jog to the right.

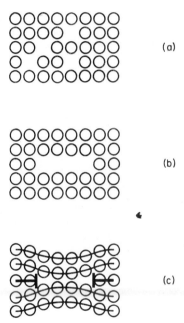

FIG. 3.15. Formation of a prismatic dislocation loop. (a) Represents a crystal
with a large non-equilibrium concentration of vacancies. In (b) the vacancies have collected on a close-packed plane and in (c) the disc has collapsed
to form an edge dislocation loop.

Secondly, a chemical force due to a deviation of the concentration
of vacancies from the equilibrium value, at the prevailing temperature, around the dislocation. If there is an excess of vacancies they
tend to combine with the dislocation at the jog to restore the
equilibrium concentration and move the jog to the left. If the net
velocity of the jogs is $v_c$, the rate of climb of the dislocation normal

to its slip plane is

$$v = v_c \frac{b}{x} \tag{3.6}$$

where $b$ is the spacing between the atom planes.

Pure screw dislocations have no extra half plane and in principle cannot climb. However, a small edge component or a jog on a screw dislocation will provide a site for the start of climb. Two examples will serve to illustrate the climb process in both edge and predominantly screw dislocations.

### 3.7 Experimental Observation of Climb

PRISMATIC DISLOCATION LOOPS

The Burgers vector of the dislocation loop in Fig. 3.8 lies in the slip plane which is also the plane of the loop. When the Burgers vector is not in the plane of the loop, the slip surface defined by the dislocation line and its Burgers vector is a cylindrical surface. The dislocation is called a *prismatic dislocation*. It follows that the dislocation can only move conservatively, i.e. by glide along the cylindrical surface and if the loop expands or shrinks *climb* must be occurring. Numerous examples of prismatic loops have been observed using transmission electron microscopy. They can be formed in the following way. The large excess concentration of vacancies resulting from rapid quenching from a high temperature (see section 1.5) may precipitate out in the form of a disc on a close-packed plane. If the disc is large enough, it is energetically favourable for it to collapse to produce a dislocation loop (Fig. 3.15). The Burgers vector of the loop is normal to the plane of the loop, so that an edge dislocation has been formed. In the presence of an excess concentration of vacancies the loops will expand by positive climb. Alternatively if there is a nearby sink for vacancies the loops will emit vacancies and shrink by *negative climb*. Figure 3.16 shows an example of the latter. The dislocation loops were formed in a thin sheet of aluminium by

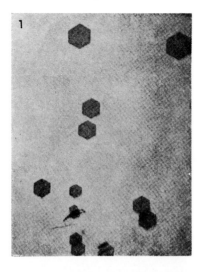

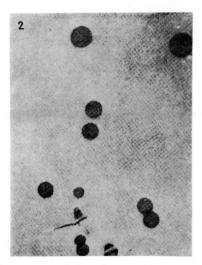

FIG. 3.16. Electron transmission photographic sequence showing the shrinkage of $\frac{1}{3} \langle 111 \rangle$ stacking fault dislocation loops in aluminium by negative climb. The foil was annealed at 102°C for 0, 213, 793 and 1301 min, respectively. (From TARTOUR and WASHBURN, *Phil. Mag.* **18**, 1257, 1968.)

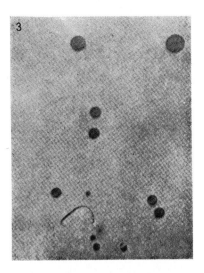

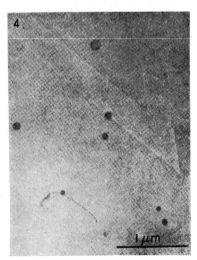

FIG. 3.16. *(cont.)*

quenching. The sheet was thinned to about 100 nm and examined by transmission electron microscopy. The surfaces of the sheet are very effective sinks for vacancies and when the foil was heated in the microscope to allow thermal activation to assist in the formation and diffusion of vacancies, the loops shrank and disappeared.

## HELICAL DISLOCATIONS

Dislocations in the form of a long spiral have been observed in crystals which have been thermally treated to produce climb conditions. Thus, in Fig. 3.17a, the helical dislocation in $CaF_2$ was formed by heating the crystal to a high temperature. The helical dislocations in Fig. 3.17b were formed by quenching the aluminium alloy from a temperature close to its melting point. A mechanism for the formation of helical dislocations has been given by Amelinckx *et al.* (1957). The dislocation $AB$, in Fig. 3.18, is pinned or locked at $A$ and $B$. The dislocation is partly edge and partly screw in character. Motion of the dislocation in the plane $ABA'$ corresponds to glide since this plane contains the line and the Burgers vector. Motion at right angles to this plane corresponds to climb. An excess of vacancies at a suitable temperature will cause the dislocation to climb. The configuration of the dislocation after a certain amount of climb is shown in Fig. 3.18(b). The dislocation now lies on the surface of a cylinder whose axis is parallel to the Burgers vector (i.e. prismatic dislocation) and it can glide on the surface of the cylinder. Further climb displaces each part of the dislocation in a direction normal to the surface of the cylinder. The dislocation will change into a double spiral as shown in Fig. 3.18(c). The radius of the spiral will be smallest at the nodes, since, for a given number of vacancies, the angle of rotation will be greater there. If $A'B$ is small compared with $AA'$, combination of prismatic glide and climb will result in the formation of a uniformly spaced spiral. The Burgers vector of the helical dislocation illustrated in Fig. 3.18 must therefore lie along the axis of the helix. The helix consists essentially of a screw dislocation parallel to the axis of the helix and a set of prismatic loops.

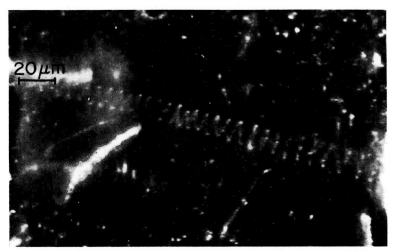

FIG. 3.17. (a) Spiral or helical dislocation in CaF$_2$ (fluorite) revealed by the decoration technique. (After BONTINCK and AMELINCKX, *Phil. Mag.* **2**, 94, 1957.)

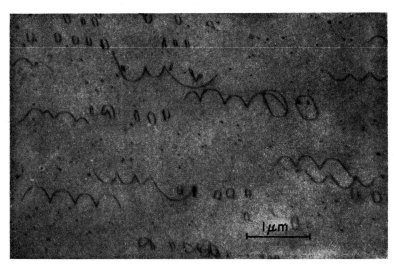

(b) Transmission electron micrograph of helical dislocations and individual dislocation loops in an aluminium 1·25 per cent silicon alloy quenched from 550°C into 50°C distilled water. (From WESTMACOTT, BARNES, HULL and SMALLMAN, *Phil. Mag.* **6**, 929, 1961.)

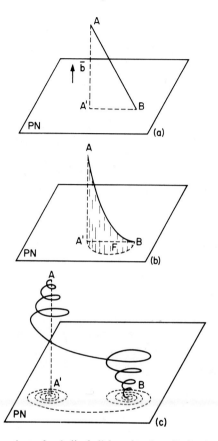

Fig. 3.18. Formation of a helical dislocation by climb of a straight dislocation with a screw component. (a) A straight dislocation line *AB* and its projection in the plane *PN* which is normal to the Burgers vector **b** and passes through *B*. *A'* is the projection of *A* on to plane *PN*. (b) Change produced in the dislocation *AB* by climb. *AB* is now curved and lies on a cylinder whose axis is parallel to **b**. The dislocation can glide on this cylinder. The area *F* is proportional to the amount of material added or lost in climb. (c) Helical dislocation produced after further climb. The projection of this dislocation on to *PN* is the double spiral shown in the diagram. (From Amelinckx, Bontinck, Dekeyser and Seitz, *Phil. Mag.* **2**, 355, 1957.)

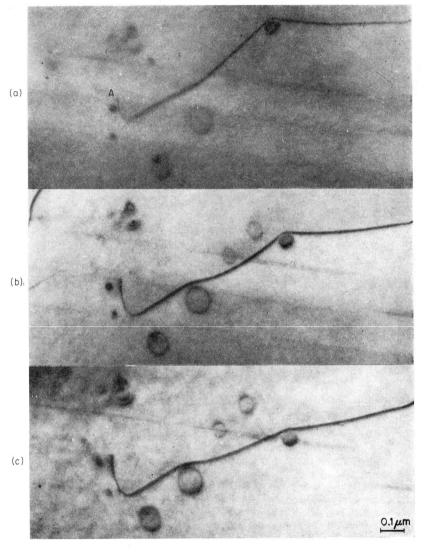

(a)

(b)

(c)

0.1 μm

FIG. 3.19. Sequence of electron micrographs showing the conservative climb motion of a dislocaton loop, with a Burgers vector normal to the plane of the loop, due to its interaction with an edge dislocation. (From KROUPA and PRICE, *Phil. Mag.* **6**, 243, 1961.)

## 3.8 Conservative Climb

From the description of the basic types of dislocation movement at the beginning of this chapter the heading of this section appears to be a contradiction. However, Kroupa and Price made the following observation: a prismatic dislocation loop (see Fig. 3.15), which can *glide* only along the cylinder contained by the dislocation line and its Burgers vector, and can *climb* only by expanding or shrinking, was observed to move under the influence of the stress field of a long edge dislocation, in the plane of the loop maintaining its original size (Fig. 3.19). This is a climb process since the dislocation moves out of its glide cylinder, but since there is no change in the size of the loop it follows that there is no net loss or gain of vacancies, i.e. no bulk diffusion has occurred. Kroupa and Price have analysed this situation in some detail and conclude that climb is occurring, not by self diffusion, but by the transfer of vacancies around the loop by *pipe diffusion*, the vacancies producing positive climb at one side of the loop and negative climb at the other side. By this mechanism the loop can move in its own plane. The process is called *conservative climb*.

*Further Reading*

The books and paper listed under "Dislocations" at the end of Chapter 1 provide excellent sources of further information.

AMELINCKX, S., BONTINCK, W., DEKEYSER, W. and SEITZ, F. (1957) "On the formation and properties of helical dislocations", *Phil. Mag.* **2**, 355.

GILMAN, J. J. (1969) *Micromechanics of Flow in Solids*, McGraw-Hill.

GILLIS, P. P., GILMAN, J. J. and TAYLOR, J. W. (1969) "Stress dependences of dislocation velocities", *Phil. Mag.* **20**, 279.

GROVES, G. W. and KELLY, A. (1969) "Change of shape due to dislocation climb", *Phil. Mag.* **19**, 977.

IMURA, T. (1972) "Dynamic studies of plastic deformation by means of high voltage electron microscopy", *Electron Microscopy and Strength of Materials*, p. 104, University of California Press.

JOHNSTON, W. G. (1962) "Yield points and delay times in single crystals", *J. Appl. Phys.* **33**, 2716.

JOHNSTON, W. G. and GILMAN, J. J. (1959) "Dislocation velocities, dislocation densities and plastic flow in lithium fluoride crystals", *J. Appl. Phys.* **30**, 129.

NIX, W. D., GASCA-NERI, R. and HIRTH, J. P. (1971) "A contribution to the theory of dislocation climb", *Phil. Mag.* **23,** 1339.

ROSENFIELD, A. R., HAHN, G. T., BEMENT, A. L. and JAFFEE, R. I. (Eds.) (1968) *Dislocation Dynamics*, McGraw-Hill.

SCHMID, E. and BOAS, W. (1950) *Plasticity of Crystals*, Hughes & Co. Ltd.

SMALLMAN, R. E. and DOBSON, P. S. (1966) "The climb of dislocation loops in zinc", *Proc. Roy. Soc.* A **293,** 423.

STEIN, D. F. and LOW, J. W. (1960) "Mobility of edge dislocations in silicon iron crystals", *J. Appl. Phys.* **31,** 362.

CHAPTER 4

# Elastic Properties of Dislocations

## 4.1 Introduction

The displacement of the lattice required to produce a dislocation results in an elastic stress field being created round the dislocation. For example, consider the edge dislocation in Fig. 1.15. The region above the slip plane, containing the extra half plane, which has been forced between the normal lattice planes, will be in compression, and the region below the slip plane will be in tension. Using the theory of elasticity a good approximation of the stress field can be obtained. The crystal is assumed to be an isotropic elastic continuum. From a knowledge of the stress field the energy of the dislocation, forces between dislocations, and similar parameters, can be obtained.

## 4.2 Nomenclature—Components of Stress

The stress at a point in a solid can be resolved into normal and shear components. The stress components can be described with respect to an elemental cube as illustrated in Fig. 4.1. The three visible faces are called the front faces and the others are called the rear faces. A shear stress can be resolved into two components in a given plane. Thus for the (100) plane the shearing stress has components $\sigma_{xz}$ and $\sigma_{xy}$. The first subscript indicates the plane in which the stress acts and the second the direction in which the stress acts.

*Introduction to Dislocations*

The plane is best defined by its normal, thus $\sigma_{xz}$ is a shear stress on a plane perpendicular to the $x$-axis in the direction of the $z$-axis. Stresses acting normal to the faces of the cube are not resolvable into two components and are described by a single subscript denoting the directions in which the stress acts; i.e. $\sigma_x$ is the normal stress acting in the $x$-direction.

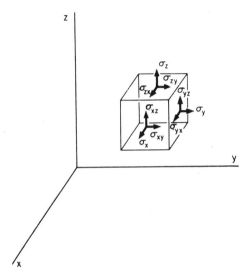

FIG. 4.1. Components of stress acting on an elemental unit cube. These correspond to the forces that are exerted on the material inside the cube by the material outside.

The stress components on the front faces are taken as positive. The stress components on the rear faces are negatives of those on the front faces. Normal tensile stresses are positive and normal compressive stresses are negative.

Nine stress components must be defined to describe the state of stress at a point, namely $\sigma_x$, $\sigma_y$, $\sigma_z$, $\sigma_{xy}$, $\sigma_{xz}$, $\sigma_{yx}$, $\sigma_{yz}$, $\sigma_{zx}$ and $\sigma_{zy}$. By considering moments of forces about the coordinate axes through the centre of the elemental cube it can be shown that for equilibrium at any point

$$\sigma_{xy} = \sigma_{yx}, \qquad \sigma_{zx} = \sigma_{xz}, \qquad \sigma_{yz} = \sigma_{zy}. \tag{4.1}$$

It is sometimes more convenient to use cylindrical coordinates of stress as illustrated in Fig. 4.2. Thus, $\sigma_r$ is the radial stress, $\sigma_\theta$ is the circumferential stress and the nine stress components are $\sigma_r$, $\sigma_\theta$, $\sigma_z$, $\sigma_{r\theta}$, $\sigma_{\theta r}$, $\sigma_{rz}$, $\sigma_{zr}$, $\sigma_{z\theta}$, $\sigma_{\theta z}$.

### 4.3 Stress Field of a Dislocation

SCREW DISLOCATION

The elastic distortion around a dislocation can be represented in terms of the deformation of a cylindrical ring of isotropic material.

Consider the screw dislocation *AB* shown in Fig. 4.2(a); the ring of isotropic material in Fig. 4.2(b) has been deformed to produce a

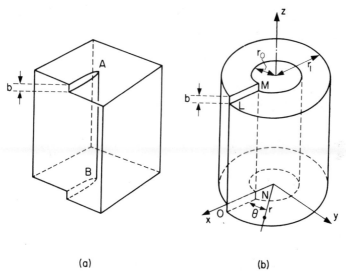

(a)                                (b)

FIG. 4.2. (a) Screw dislocation *AB* formed in a crystal. (b) Elastic distortion of a cylindrical ring simulating the distortion produced by the screw dislocation *AB*.

similar distortion. A radial slit *LMNO* was cut in the ring parallel to the *z*-axis and then the free surfaces were displaced rigidly with respect to each other by the distance $b$, the magnitude of the Burgers vector of the screw dislocation, in the $z$-direction. A uniform shear strain $\varepsilon_{\theta z}$ ( $= \varepsilon_{z\theta}$) is produced throughout the ring which is equal to the step height $b$ divided by the circumference $2\pi r$, of a cylindrical element, radius $r$,

$$\varepsilon_{\theta z} = \frac{b}{2\pi r} . \tag{4.2}$$

The corresponding stress

$$\sigma_{\theta z} = \sigma_{z\theta} = \frac{Gb}{2\pi r} \tag{4.3}$$

where $G$ is the shear modulus. Since the displacement of the ring is produced by a shear in the $z$-direction there will be no displacements in the $x$- and $y$-directions and the other stress components will be zero

$$\sigma_r = \sigma_\theta = \sigma_z = \sigma_{r\theta} = \sigma_{\theta r} = \sigma_{rz} = \sigma_{zr} = 0. \tag{4.4}$$

Thus the stress field consists of two pure shears; $\sigma_{\theta z}$ in radial planes parallel to the $z$-direction and $\sigma_{z\theta}$ in planes normal to the $z$-axis perpendicular to the radius.

The stress field has radial symmetry around the dislocation, i.e. $\sigma_{\theta z} = Gb/2\pi r$ and is independent of $\theta$. This is closely related to the fact that a screw dislocation has no extra half plane and cannot be identified with a particular slip plane.

In rectangular coordinates the components of stress of a screw dislocation are

$$\sigma_{xz} = \sigma_{zx} = -\frac{Gb}{2\pi} \frac{y}{x^2 + y^2} ,$$

$$\sigma_{yz} = \sigma_{zy} = \frac{Gb}{2\pi} \frac{x}{x^2 + y^2} , \tag{4.5}$$

$$\sigma_x = \sigma_y = \sigma_z = \sigma_{xy} = \sigma_{yx} = 0.$$

## Edge Dislocation

The stress field is more complex than that of a screw but can be represented in an isotropic ring in a similar way. Considering the edge dislocation in Fig. 4.3(a), the same elastic strain field can be produced in the ring by a rigid displacement of the faces of the slit by a distance $b$ in the $x$-direction (Fig. 4.3(b)). The strains in the

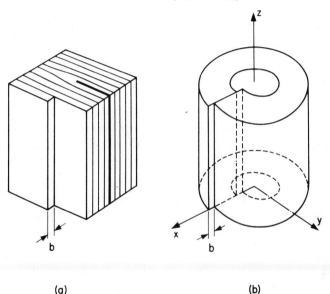

(a)                                           (b)

Fig. 4.3. (a) Edge dislocation formed in a crystal. (b) Elastic distortion of a cylindrical ring simulating the distortion produced by the edge dislocation in (a).

$z$-direction are zero and the deformation is basically plane strain. The stress components determined using isotropic theory are

$$\sigma_x = -Dy\,\frac{(3x^2+y^2)}{(x^2+y^2)^2}$$

$$\sigma_y = Dy\,\frac{(x^2-y^2)}{(x^2+y^2)^2}$$

$$\sigma_{xy} = \sigma_{yx} = Dx \frac{(x^2 - y^2)}{(x^2 + y^2)^2} \qquad (4.6)$$

$$\sigma_z = \nu(\sigma_x + \sigma_y)$$

$$\sigma_{xz} = \sigma_{zx} = \sigma_{yz} = \sigma_{zy} = 0$$

where
$$D = \frac{Gb}{2\pi(1 - \nu)}$$

and $\nu$ is Poisson's ratio. The stress field has, therefore, both dilational and shear components. The largest normal stress is $\sigma_x$ which acts parallel to the slip vector. Since the slip plane can be defined as $y = 0$, the maximum compressive stress ($\sigma_x$ is negative) acts immediately above the slip plane and the maximum tensile stress ($\sigma_x$ is positive) acts immediately below the slip plane. This observation is implied qualitatively by the type of distortion illustrated in Fig. 1.15.

The equations listed above have been used widely in studying dislocation problems. There are a number of limitations which must be realised. Firstly, the elastic solutions apply to a *ring* of isotropic material and not to a *solid* cylinder. Equations (4.3) and (4.6) show that the stress varies inversely with distance from the centre of ring, i.e. as $1/r$, and therefore it will rise to infinity at $r = 0$. Clearly infinite stresses cannot be supported at the centre of a dislocation and there is a limiting radius $r_o$ below which the elastic solutions do not apply. Estimates of $r_o$ suggest that it is of the order of 1 nm. The central region around the dislocation, radius $r_o$, is referred to as the *core of the dislocation*. Secondly, a real crystal is not an isotropic continuum and in the core of the dislocation it is necessary to consider the displacements of, and forces between, individual atoms. These provide very difficult mathematical problems and the properties of the core are, at present, not well understood.

### 4.4 Strain Energy of a Dislocation

The existence of an elastically distorted region around a dislocation implies that a body containing a dislocation has an extra strain energy.

The total strain energy may be divided into two parts

$$E_{\text{total}} = E_{\text{core}} + E_{\text{elastic strain}}. \tag{4.7}$$

The amount of elastic energy stored in the crystal may be obtained by calculating the work done by the forces acting on the cut faces (see Figs. 4.2 and 4.3) in displacing them a distance $b$ to form the dislocation. Alternatively, the elastic strain energy may be determined by integration of the energy stored in each small element of volume. This is a simple calculation for screw dislocations. The element of volume is a cylindrical shell of radius $r$ and thickness $dr$. The shear strain in this element is constant, $\varepsilon_{\theta z} = b/2\pi r$, equation (4.2). Since the strain is linear and elastic the energy will be $\frac{1}{2}$x (elastic modulus) x (strain)$^2$, per unit volume and the strain energy stored in the element will be

$$dE_{\text{el}(S)} = \tfrac{1}{2} G(\varepsilon_{\theta z})^2 \, 2\pi r \, dr \tag{4.8}$$

per unit length, and the elastic strain energy per unit length of screw dislocation in the region from the core to the radius $R$ is

$$E_{\text{el}(S)} = \frac{1}{2} \int_{r_0}^{R} \frac{Gb^2}{2\pi r} \, dr$$

or

$$E_{\text{el}(S)} = \frac{Gb^2}{4\pi} \ln \left( \frac{R}{r_0} \right). \tag{4.9}$$

If $R$ is taken to be the external diameter of the crystal it follows that the elastic energy in a crystal containing a single dislocation will depend on the size of the crystal. The corresponding equation for the strain energy of an edge dislocation is

$$E_{\text{el}(E)} = \frac{Gb^2}{4\pi(1-\nu)} \ln \left( \frac{R}{r_0} \right). \tag{4.10}$$

Thus, the elastic energy of an edge dislocation is more than that of the screw dislocation by $1/(1-\nu)$. Taking $R = 1$ mm, $r_0 = 1$ nm, $G = 40$ GN m$^{-2}$, and $b = 0.25$ nm the elastic strain energy of an edge dislocation will be about 4 nJ m$^{-1}$ (4×10$^{-4}$ erg cm$^{-1}$) or about 1 aJ (6 eV) for each atom plane threaded by the dislocation.

In crystals containing many dislocations, the elastic stress fields of adjacent dislocations tend to cancel each other. The appropriate value of $R$ is usually taken as half the average spacing of the dislocations arranged at random.

Estimates of the energy of the core of the dislocation are necessarily very approximate. However, the estimates that have been made suggest that the core energy will be of the order of 0·1–0·3 aJ for each atom plane threaded by the dislocation which is only a small fraction of the elastic energy.

However, in contrast to the elastic energy, the energy of the core will vary as the dislocation moves through the crystal and this gives rise to the lattice resistance to dislocation motion  discussed in section 10.2.

It was mentioned in section 3.3 that most dislocations have a *mixed edge-screw character*. To calculate the energy of such dislocations they may be considered as two superimposed dislocations as illustrated in Fig. 3.7(b). The Burgers vector of the mixed dislocation **b** is resolved into an edge dislocation **b**$_1$ and a screw dislocation **b**$_2$ where $b_1 = b \sin \theta$ and $b_2 = b \cos \theta$. Since the Burgers vectors of these dislocations are at right angles there will be no elastic energy associated with the interaction between the dislocation (section 4.6) and the total elastic energy will be the sum of the self-energies of edge and screw dislocations (equations (4.9) and (4.10)). Thus

$$E_{\text{el}(M)} = \left\{ \frac{Gb^2 \sin^2 \theta}{4\pi(1-\nu)} + \frac{Gb^2 \cos^2 \theta}{4\pi} \right\} \left[ \ln \left( \frac{R}{r_0} \right) \right]$$

$$= \frac{Gb^2}{4\pi(1-\nu)} \ln \left( \frac{R}{r_0} \right) [1 - \nu \cos^2 \theta], \qquad (4.11)$$

which is somewhere between the energy of an edge and a screw dislocation.

From the expressions for edge, screw and mixed dislocations it is clear that the energy per unit length is relatively insensitive to the character of the dislocation and also to the values of $R$ and $r_0$. Taking realistic values for $R$ and $r_0$ all the equations can be written approximately as

$$E_{el} = \alpha G b^2 \qquad (4.12)$$

where $\alpha \approx 0 \cdot 5 - 1 \cdot 0$. This leads to a very simple rule (Frank rule) for determining whether or not a dislocation reaction will occur (for more details, see Chapter 7). Consider the reaction of two $\frac{1}{2}\langle 111 \rangle$ slip dislocations in a body-centred cubic metal moving in two different slip planes and interacting to produce a third dislocation

$$\left. \begin{array}{c} \frac{1}{2}[1\bar{1}\bar{1}] + \frac{1}{2}[111] \rightarrow [100], \\ \mathbf{b}_1 + \mathbf{b}_2 \rightarrow \mathbf{b}. \end{array} \right\} \qquad (4.13)$$

From equation (4.12) the elastic strain energies of these dislocations are proportional to $b_1^2$, $b_2^2$ and $b^2$. Since $b_1^2 = a^2(\frac{1}{4} + \frac{1}{4} + \frac{1}{4})$ $b_2^2 = a^2(\frac{1}{4} + \frac{1}{4} + \frac{1}{4})$ and $b^2 = a^2(1 + 0 + 0)$, it follows that when the dislocations meet the reaction results in a reduction in energy, and therefore tends to occur. In the more general case a dislocation of strength $b$ will tend to dissociate into dislocations $b_1$ and $b_2$ when $b^2 > b_1^2 + b_2^2$. In this argument the assumption is made that there is no additional interaction energy involved, i.e. that before and after the reaction the reacting dislocations are separated sufficiently so that the interaction energy is small.

## 4.5 Forces on Dislocations

When a sufficiently high stress is applied to a crystal containing dislocations, the dislocations move and produce plastic deformation by slip. The applied stress therefore does work on the crystal through the movement of dislocations and consequently there is effectively a *force* acting on a dislocation line causing it to move forward. Consider a dislocation moving in a slip plane under the influence of a uniform shear stress (Fig. 4.4). When an element d$s$ of the dislocation line Burgers vector $\mathbf{b}$ moves forward a distance d$l$ the crystal above and below the slip plane will be displaced relative to each other. The

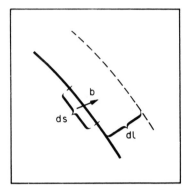

FIG. 4.4. Force acting on a dislocation line.

average shear displacement produced is

$$\left(\frac{\mathrm{d}s\,\mathrm{d}l}{A}\right)b \tag{4.14}$$

where $A$ is the area of the slip plane. The applied force giving the stress $\tau$ is $A\tau$ so that the work done when the element of slip occurs is

$$\mathrm{d}W = A\tau\left(\frac{\mathrm{d}s\,\mathrm{d}l}{A}\right)b. \tag{4.15}$$

*The force F on a unit length of dislocation is defined as the work done when unit length of dislocation moves unit distance.* Therefore

$$F = \frac{\mathrm{d}W}{\mathrm{d}s\,\mathrm{d}l} = \frac{\mathrm{d}W}{\mathrm{d}A} = \tau b. \tag{4.16}$$

The force is normal to the dislocation at every point along its length and is directed towards the unslipped part of the glide plane.

In addition to the force due to an externally applied stress, a dislocation has a *line tension* which is analogous to the surface tension of a soap bubble or a liquid. This arises because, as outlined in the previous section, the strain energy of a dislocation is proportional to its length and any increase in length results in an increase in energy. The

line tension has units of energy per unit length. From the approximation used in equation (4.12), the line tension, which may be defined
as *the increase in energy per unit increase in the length of a dislocation
line*, will be

$$T = \alpha G b^2 \tag{4.17}$$

Consider the curved dislocation in Fig. 4.5. The line tension will
produce a force tending to straighten the line and so reduce the total
energy of the line. The direction of the force is perpendicular to the
dislocation and towards the centre of curvature. The line will only
remain curved if there is a shear stress which produces a force on the

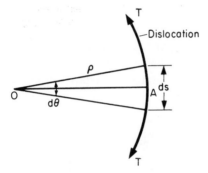

FIG. 4.5. Line tension of a dislocation.

dislocation line in the opposite sense. The shear stress $\tau_0$ needed to
maintain a radius of curvature $\varrho$ is found in the following way. Consider an elementary arc $ds$ of a dislocation line. The angle subtended
at the centre of curvature is $d\theta = ds/\varrho$. The outward force along $OA$
due to the applied stress acting on the elementary piece of dislocation
is $\tau_0 b \, ds$, and the opposing inward force along $OA$ due to the line
tension $T$ at the ends of the element is $2T \sin (d\theta/2)$ which is equal to
$T d\theta$ for small values of $d\theta$. The line will be in equilibrium in this curved
position when

$$T \, d\theta = \tau_0 b \, ds,$$

$$\tau_0 = \frac{T}{b\varrho} . \tag{4.18}$$

Substituting for $T$ from equation (4.17)

$$\tau_0 = \frac{\alpha Gb}{\varrho}.\qquad(4.19)$$

This gives an expression for the stress required to bend a dislocation to a radius $\varrho$ and is used many times in subsequent chapters. A particularly direct application is in the understanding of the Frank–Read dislocation multiplication source described in Chapter 8.

### 4.6 Forces between Dislocations

A simple semi-qualitative argument will illustrate the significance of the concept of a force between dislocations. Consider two parallel edge dislocations lying in the same slip plane. They can either have the same sign as in Fig. 4.6(a) or opposite sign as in Fig. 4.6(b). When the dislocations are separated by a large distance the total elastic energy of the dislocations in both situations will be

$$2\frac{Gb^2}{4\pi(1-\nu)}\ln\left(\frac{R}{r_0}\right)\qquad(4.20)$$

assuming that all the dislocations are of unit length. When the dislocations in Fig. 4.6(a) are very close together the arrangement can be considered approximately as a single dislocation with a Burgers vector magnitude $2b$ and the elastic energy will be given by

$$\frac{G(2b)^2}{4\pi(1-\nu)}\ln\left(\frac{R}{r_0}\right)\qquad(4.21)$$

which is twice the energy of the dislocations when they are separated by a large distance. Thus the dislocations will tend to repel each other to reduce their total elastic energy. When dislocations of opposite sign (Fig. 4.6(b)) are close together, the effective magnitude of their Burgers vectors will be zero, and the corresponding long-range elastic energy, zero also. Thus dislocations of opposite sign will attract each other to reduce their total elastic energy. The positive and negative edge dislocations in Fig. 4.6(b) will combine and annihilate each other. An interesting possibility exists when the two dislocations lie on slip planes separated by a few atomic distances as in Fig. 4.6(c). The dislocations cannot annihilate each other completely to form a region of perfect lattice. However, they may combine to form a row of vacancies (Fig. 4.6(d)) or interstitial atoms.

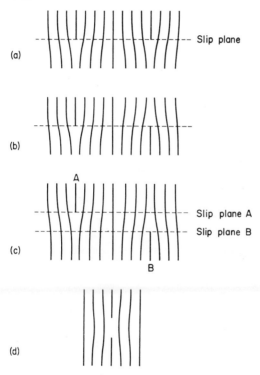

FIG. 4.6. Arrangement of edge dislocations with parallel Burgers vectors lying in parallel slip planes. (a) like dislocations on the same slip plane, (b) unlike dislocations on the same slip plane, (c) unlike dislocations on slip planes separated by a few atomic spacings, (d) combination of the dislocations in (c) to form a row of vacancies.

The magnitude of the force between dislocations has been calculated for a few simple dislocation arrangements. The basis of the

method used is to determine the work done in introducing a dislocation into a crystal which already contains a dislocation. Consider two
edge dislocations (Fig. 4.7) lying parallel to the $z$-axis with parallel
Burgers vectors in the $x$-direction. The total energy of the system can
be divided into three parts, (1) self-energy of dislocation $I$, (2) self-
energy of dislocation $II$, and (3) interaction energy between $I$ and $II$.
The interaction energy is obtained from the total work done in intro-

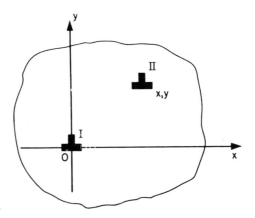

FIG. 4.7. Interaction between two edge dislocations. (After COTTRELL
(1953), *Dislocations and Plastic Flow in Crystals*, Oxford University Press.)

ducing $II$ into the crystal at the position $(x, y)$ by subtracting the self-
energy of $II$. The force will be obtained by differentiation since from
equation (4.16) $F = \mathrm{d}W/\mathrm{d}A$ for a unit length of dislocation line. The
results obtained are as follows: the force per unit length is given by
the following components,

$$\left.\begin{array}{l} F_x = \sigma_{xy}b, \\ F_y = \sigma_x b, \end{array}\right\} \tag{4.22}$$

where $F_x$ is the force component in the common glide direction and
$F_y$ the force component perpendicular to the glide plane. Substituting

equation (4.6)

$$F_x = \frac{Gb^2}{2\pi(1-\nu)} \frac{x(x^2-y^2)}{(x^2+y^2)^2}$$

$$F_y = -\frac{Gb^2}{2\pi(1-\nu)} \frac{y(3x^2+y^2)}{(x^2+y^2)^2} \,,$$

(4.23)

Since edge dislocations can move by slip only in the plane contained by the dislocation line and its Burgers vector the component of force which is most important in determining the behaviour of the dislocations in Fig. 4.7 is $F_x$. Thus $F_x$ is positive for two dislocations of the same sign for all values of $x > y$ and the dislocations will repel each other. For dislocations of opposite sign, $F_x$ will be positive for $x > y$ and the dislocations will attract each other. In Fig. 4.8 the force is

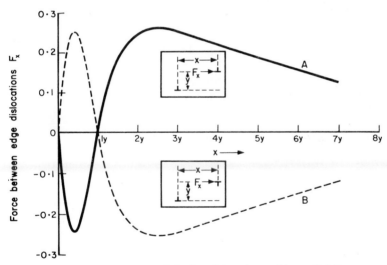

FIG. 4.8. Force between parallel edge dislocations with parallel Burgers vectors from equation (4.23). Unit of force $F_x$ is

$$\frac{Gb^2}{2\pi(1-\nu)\,y} \cdot$$

The full curve $A$ is for like dislocations, and the broken curve $B$ for unlike dislocations. (After COTTRELL (1953) *Dislocations and Plastic Flow in Crystals*, Oxford University Press.)

plotted against distance apart, $x$, expressed in units of $y$. The full curve $A$ is for like dislocations and the broken curve $B$ is for unlike dislocations. $F_x$ is zero at $x = 0$ and $x = y$. It follows that an array of edge dislocations of the same sign is most stable when the dislocations lie vertically above one another. This is the arrangement of dislocations in a small angle pure tilt boundary described in Chapter 9.

The forces between parallel screw dislocations are simpler than those between edge dislocations because the stress field of a screw dislocation has radial symmetry. Consider two screw dislocations lying parallel to the $z$-axis. The only component of force acts along the line joining the dislocations in the plane $z = $ constant, thus

$$F_r = \sigma_{\theta z} b \qquad (4.24)$$

and substituting from equation (4.3)

$$F_r = \frac{Gb^2}{2\pi r} . \qquad (4.25)$$

The force is attractive for dislocations of opposite sign and repulsive for dislocations of the same sign.

*Further Reading*

COTTRELL, A. H. (1953) *Dislocations and Plastic Flow in Crystals*, Oxford University Press.

FRIEDEL, J. (1964) *Dislocations*, Pergamon Press.

HIRTH, J. P. and LOTHE, J. (1968) *Theory of Dislocations*, McGraw-Hill.

NABARRO, F. R. N. (1967) *The Theory of Crystal Dislocations*, Oxford University. Press.

SEEGER, A. (1955) "Theory of lattice imperfections", *Handbuch der Physik*, Vol. VII, part 1, p. 383, Springer-Verlag.

SIMMONS, J. A., DE WIT, R. and BULLOUGH, R. (Eds.) (1970) *Fundamental Aspects of Dislocation Theory*, National Bureau of Standards.

WEERTMAN, J. and WEERTMAN, J. R. (1964) *Elementary Dislocation Theory*, Macmillan.

CHAPTER 5

# Dislocations in Face-centred Cubic Crystals

## 5.1 Unit Dislocations

Many common metals such as copper, silver, gold, aluminium, nickel and their alloys, have a face-centred cubic structure. The pure metals are soft and ductile but they can be hardened considerably by plastic deformation and alloying. The deformation behaviour is closely related to the structure of the dislocations which is more complex than that described in Chapter 1 for the simple cubic structure.

The principal lattice vectors, and therefore the most likely Burgers vectors for dislocations in the face-centred cubic structure, are of the type $\frac{1}{2}\langle 110 \rangle$ and $\langle 001 \rangle$. Since the energy of a dislocation is proportional to the square of the magnitude of its Burgers vector, $b^2$ (section 4.4), the energy of $\frac{1}{2}\langle 110 \rangle$ dislocations will be only half that of $\langle 001 \rangle$, i.e. $2a^2/4$ compared with $a^2$. Thus, $\langle 001 \rangle$ dislocations are much less favoured energetically, and, in fact, have not been observed. Figure 5.1 represents a $\frac{1}{2}\langle 110 \rangle$ edge dislocation in a face-centred cubic lattice. The "extra half plane" consists of two (110) planes which occur in an $ABAB\ldots$ sequence. There is one $A$ layer and one $B$ layer. Movement of this unit dislocation by glide involves a successive displacement such that the unit $A+B$ configuration is retained.

## 5.2 Partial Dislocations—the Shockley Partial

Examination of Fig. 5.1 suggests that the two extra (110) planes
will tend to move independently and this is described in section 5.3.
The independent movement requires displacements less than a unit
lattice vector and occurs by the movement of *partial dislocations*.

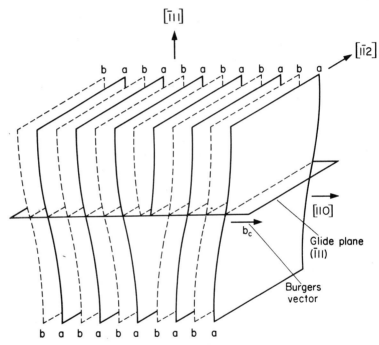

FIG. 5.1. Unit edge dislocation $\frac{1}{2}$[110] in a face-centred cubic crystal.
(From SEEGER (1957), *Dislocations and Mechanical Properties of Crystals*,
p. 243, Wiley.)

When a stacking fault ends inside a crystal, the boundary in the
plane of the fault, separating the faulted region from the perfect region
of the crystal, is a partial dislocation. Two important partial dislocations have been recognised in face-centred cubic metals, namely
the *Shockley partial* which is associated with slip, and the *Frank*

*partial* (see section 5.5). The formation of a Shockley partial edge dislocation is illustrated in Fig. 5.2 and can be compared with the formation of a unit edge dislocation in a simple cubic lattice (Fig.

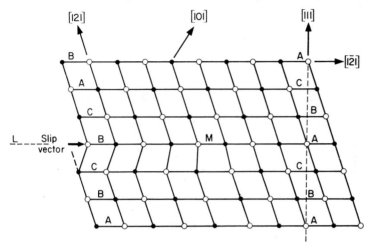

FIG. 5.2. Formation of an $\frac{1}{6}[1\bar{2}1]$ Shockley partial dislocation at $M$ due to slip along $LM$. The open circles represent the positions of atoms in the $(10\bar{1})$ plane of the diagram and the closed circles the positions of the atoms in the $(10\bar{1})$ planes immediately above and below the plane of the diagram.
(From READ (1953), *Dislocations in Crystals*, McGraw-Hill.)

3.3). The diagram represents a $(10\bar{1})$ section through the lattice. The close-packed (111) planes lie at right angles to the plane of the diagram. At the right of the diagram the $A$ layers rest on $C$ layers and the lattice is perfect. At the left of the diagram the $A$ layers along $LM$ have slipped in a $[1\bar{2}1]$ direction to a $B$ layer position, and have produced a stacking fault and a partial dislocation. The slip vector which is in the slip plane is $\mathbf{b} = \frac{1}{6}[1\bar{2}1]$, and the magnitude of the vector is $a\sqrt{6}$.

The Burgers vector of a partial dislocation is described in the same way as that of a perfect dislocation, except that the Burgers circuit must start and finish in the surface of the stacking fault; if the circuit started at any other position it would be necessary to cross the fault plane and the one-to-one correspondence of the circuits in the perfect and imperfect lattices would not be maintained. Since the Burgers vector of a partial dislocation is not a unit lattice vector, the final position of the circuit in the perfect lattice (Fig. 1.14(b)) is not a lattice site.

## 5.3 Slip

Slip occurs in close-packed {111} planes and the observed slip direction is ⟨110⟩. Since slip involves the sliding of close-packed planes of atoms over each other, a simple experiment can be made to see how this can occur. The close-packed planes can be simulated by a set of hard spheres, as illustrated schematically in Fig. 5.3.

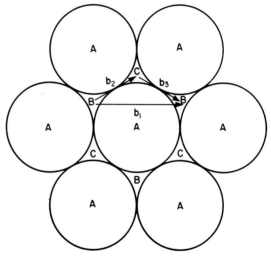

Fig. 5.3. Slip in face-centred cubic crystals. (From Cottrell (1953), *Dislocations and Plastic Flow in Crystals*, Oxford University Press.)

One layer is represented by the full circles, $A$, and the second layer rests in the sites marked $B$. Consider the movement of the layers when they are sheared over each other to produce a displacement in the slip direction. It will be found that the $B$ layer of atoms, instead of moving from one $B$ site to the next $B$ site over the top of the $A$ atoms, will move first to the nearby $C$ site along the "valley" between the two $A$ atoms and then to the new $B$ site via a second valley. Thus, the $B$ plane will slide over the $A$ plane in a zig-zag motion. In other words, the unit lattice displacement $\mathbf{b}_1$ is achieved by two movements represented by vectors $\mathbf{b}_2$ and $\mathbf{b}_3$. In terms of a moving unit $\frac{1}{2}[1\bar{1}0]$ dislocation, this demonstration suggests that it will be energetically more favourable for the $B$ atoms to move via the $C$ positions. This implies that two dislocations pass, one immediately after the other. The first has a Burgers vector $\mathbf{b}_2$ and the second a Burgers vector $\mathbf{b}_3$. The unit dislocation with Burgers vector $\mathbf{b}_1$ therefore *splits up* or *dissociates* into two dislocations $\mathbf{b}_2$ and $\mathbf{b}_3$ according to the reaction:

$$\mathbf{b}_1 \rightarrow \mathbf{b}_2 + \mathbf{b}_3 \tag{5.1}$$

or
$$\frac{1}{2}[110] \rightarrow \frac{1}{6}[211] + \frac{1}{6}[12\bar{1}]. \tag{5.2}$$

It is necessary in any proposed dislocation reaction to ensure that the sum of the components of the Burgers vectors on both sides of the reaction is the same. For reaction (5.2)

$$\frac{1}{2}[110] \rightarrow \frac{1}{6}[2+1, \, 1+2, \, 1+\bar{1}] = \frac{1}{2}[110]. \tag{5.3}$$

Since the vectors $\mathbf{b}_2$ and $\mathbf{b}_3$ are not at right angles the partial dislocations will repel each other (Chapter 4) with a force due to the elastic interaction. The force is given approximately by (Cottrell 1953),

$$F = \frac{G(\mathbf{b}_2 \cdot \mathbf{b}_3)}{2\pi d} \tag{5.4}$$

where $\mathbf{b}_2 \cdot \mathbf{b}_3$ is the scalar product of the Burgers vectors and $d$ is the distance between them. However, $\mathbf{b}_2$ and $\mathbf{b}_3$ correspond to Shockley partial dislocations and it follows that if they separate there will be a *ribbon* of stacking fault between them. The stacking sequence outside the dislocation will be $ABCABCABC$ ... and between the partial dislocations $ABCACABC$ ... The region of the fault can be regarded as a layer of twinned material and has a characteristic energy, called the *stacking fault energy* $\gamma$ which provides a force tending to pull the dislocations together. An equilibrium separation will be established when the repulsive and attractive forces balance. The equilibrium separation is obtained by equating $\gamma$ to $F$ in equation (5.4).

$$d = \frac{G(\mathbf{b}_2 \cdot \mathbf{b}_3)}{2\pi\gamma} . \tag{5.5}$$

The unit edge dislocation illustrated in Fig. 5.1 will split up as illustrated in Fig. 5.4. The configuration is called an *extended disloca-*

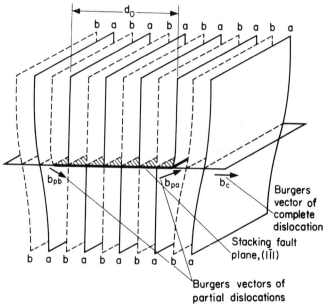

FIG. 5.4. Formation of an extended dislocation by dissociation of a unit edge dislocation (Fig. 5.1) into two Shockley partials, Burgers vectors $\mathbf{b}_{pb}$ and $\mathbf{b}_{pa}$ separated by a stacking fault. (From SEEGER (1957), *Dislocations and Mechanical Properties of Crystals*, p. 243, Wiley.)

*tion*. The width, $d$, depends on the stacking fault energy. Numerous estimates of $\gamma$ have been made and it is probable that $\gamma \approx 140$ mJ m$^{-2}$ (ergs cm$^{-2}$) for aluminium and $\gamma \approx 80$ mJ m$^{-2}$ for copper. The corresponding widths of the dislocation ribbons are about 2 and 4 Burgers vectors respectively. A fairly accurate method of determin-

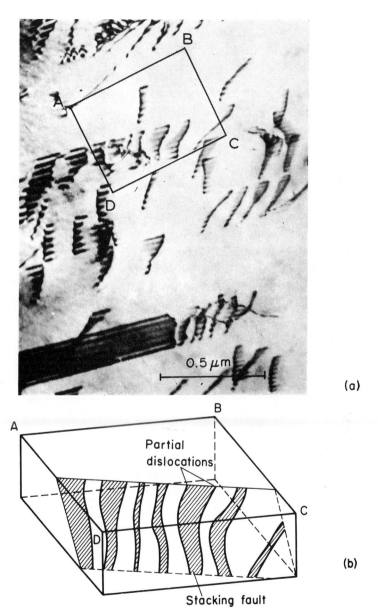

(a)

(b)

Fig. 5.5. (a) Transmission electron micrograph of extended dislocations in a copper–7 per cent aluminium alloy. (From Howie, *Metallurgical Reviews*, **6**, 467, 1961). (b) Arrangement of dislocations in the inset in (a).

ing $\gamma$, when it is small, is described in section 7.9. Frank's rule (Chapter 4) can be used to show that the dissociation (relation 5.2) is energetically favourable. Thus $b_1^2 = a^2/2$ which is greater than $b_2^2 + b_3^2 = a^2/3$.

Dissociation of unit dislocations is independent of the character (edge, screw or mixed) of the dislocation. Screw dislocations can form a similar configuration to Fig. 5.4. Unlike the unextended screw dislocation, the extended dislocation defines a specific slip plane, the $\{111\}$ plane of the fault, and will be constrained to move in this plane. The partial dislocations tend to move as a unit maintaining the equilibrium ribbon width. Experimental observations of extended dislocations in thin foils have confirmed that the dislocation geometry described above is correct. Figure 5.5 shows a set of extended dislocations lying in the same slip plane. The stacking fault between the two partials appears as a parallel fringe pattern. The individual partials are not always visible and their positions are illustrated in Fig. 5.5(b).

Although extended screw dislocations cannot cross slip (see section 3.4) it is possible to form a constriction in the screw dislocation and then the unit dislocation at the constriction will be free to move

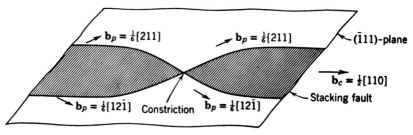

FIG. 5.6. Constriction in an extended dislocation. The drawing corresponds to a screw dislocation in a face-centred cubic lattice. (From SEEGER (1957), *Dislocations and Mechanical Properties of Crystals*, p. 243, Wiley.)

in other planes. A constriction is illustrated in Fig. 5.6. A certain amount of energy is associated with the formation of the constriction and it will form more readily in metals with a high stacking fault

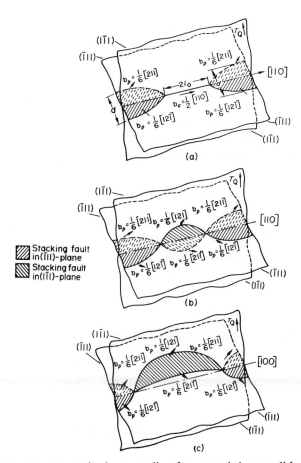

FIG. 5.7. Three stages in the cross slip of an extended screw dislocation from a ($\bar{1}$11) plane to a (1$\bar{1}$1) plane. (a) The partial dislocations have been brought together over a length $2l_0$ to form an unextended dislocation. (b) The unextended dislocation spreads out into the cross slip (1$\bar{1}$1) plane as a new extended dislocation. (c) The extended dislocation bows out in the (1$\bar{1}$1) plane between the two constrictions under the action of a shear stress $\tau_Q$. (From SEEGER (1957), *Dislocations and Mechanical Properties of Crystals*, p. 243, Wiley.)

energy such as aluminium. It follows that cross slip will be most difficult in metals with a low stacking fault energy and this produces significant effects on the deformation behaviour. Formation of a constriction can be assisted by thermal activation and hence the ease of cross slip decreases with decreasing temperature.

The sequence of events envisaged during the cross-slip process is illustrated in Fig. 5.7. An extended $\frac{1}{2}[110]$ dislocation, lying in the $(\bar{1}11)$ slip plane, has constricted along a short length $2l_0$ parallel to the [110] direction. The constricted dislocation has a pure screw orientation. A constriction is likely to form at some local region in the crystal, such as a barrier provided by non-glissile dislocations, so that the applied stress tends to push the partials together. In Fig. 5.7(b) the unit dislocation has dissociated into two different partial dislocations with a stacking fault lying in the (111) plane. This plane intersects the original glide plane along [110] and is therefore a possible cross-slip plane. The new extended dislocation is free to glide in the cross-slip plane and in Fig. 5.7(c) has bowed out between the constrictions.

### 5.4 Thompson's Tetrahedron

Thompson's tetrahedron (Thompson, 1953) is a convenient notation for describing all the important dislocations and dislocation reactions in face-centred cubic metals. It arose from the appreciation that the four different sets of {111} planes lie parallel to the four faces of a regular tetrahedron. The edges of the tetrahedron are parallel to the ⟨110⟩ slip directions, and the ribbons of stacking fault of extended dislocations will be confined to the {111} faces. The corners of the tetrahedron (Fig. 5.8) are denoted by $A$, $B$, $C$, $D$, and the mid-points of the opposite faces by $\alpha$, $\beta$, $\gamma$, $\delta$. The Burgers vectors of dislocations are specified by their two end points on the tetrahedron. Thus, the Burgers vectors of the unit dislocations are defined both in magnitude and direction by the edges of the tetrahedron and will be **AB**, **BC**, etc. Similarly, Shockley partial dislocations can be represented by the line from the corner to the centre of a face as **Aβ**, **Aγ**, etc. The disso-

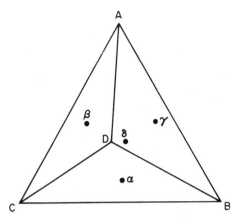

FIG. 5.8. Thompson's reference tetrahedron.

ciation of a $\frac{1}{2}\langle 110 \rangle$ dislocation described by relation (5.2) can be expressed alternatively by a reaction of the type:

$$\mathbf{AB} = \mathbf{A\delta} + \mathbf{\delta B}. \tag{5.6}$$

### 5.5 Frank Partial or Sessile Dislocation

There is an alternative arrangement by which a stacking fault can end in a crystal. Geometrically the *Frank partial dislocation* is formed by inserting or removing one close-packed layer of atoms as illustrated in Fig. 5.9. Removal of a layer results in a stacking sequence *ABCACABC* ... The boundary between the fault and the perfect crystal is a partial dislocation. The Burgers vector is normal to the {111} plane of the fault and the magnitude of the vector is equal to the change in spacing produced by one close-packed layer, i.e. $\mathbf{b} = \frac{1}{3}\langle 111 \rangle$. In Thompson's notation $\mathbf{b} = \mathbf{A\alpha}$ for a stacking fault in plane $\alpha$. The Frank partial is an edge dislocation and since the Burgers vector is not contained in a close-packed plane it cannot glide and will not move conservatively under the action of an applied stress. Such a dislocation is said to be *sessile*. However, it can move by *climb*.

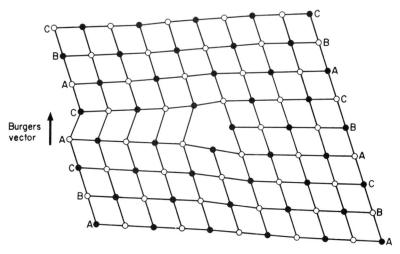

FIG. 5.9. Formation of an $\frac{1}{3}$[111] Frank partial dislocation by removal of a close-packed layer of atoms. (From READ (1953), *Dislocation in Crystals*, McGraw-Hill.)

A closed dislocation loop of a Frank partial dislocation can be produced by the collapse of a platelet of vacancies as illustrated in Fig. 3.15 (an excess concentration of vacancies is produced by rapid quenching, see section 1.5). By convention this is called a *negative Frank sessile dislocation*. A *positive Frank sessile dislocation* may be formed by the precipitation of a close-packed platelet of interstitial atoms (these can be produced by irradiation with energetic atomic particles). In both positive and negative Frank sessile dislocation loops stacking faults are produced. Diffraction fringes due to stacking faults (section 2.4) are sometimes observed when dislocation loops, produced by quenching, are examined in the electron microscope. An example is given in Fig. 5.10(a); this shows an hexagonal loop formed in an aluminium alloy containing 3·5 per cent magnesium. The sides of the loop are parallel to ⟨110⟩ close-packed directions in the fault plane. In most cases no stacking fault contrast is observed (Fig. 3.17(b)). The stacking fault can be removed by a dislocation reaction involving the stacking fault and the Frank

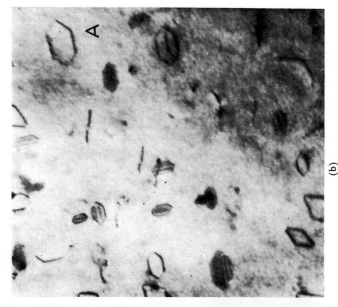

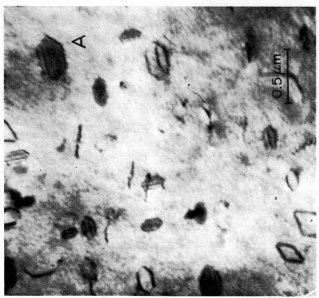

(a)        (b)

FIG. 5.10. Prismatic and sessile dislocation loops in an aluminium 3·5 per cent magnesium alloy quenched from 550°C into silicone oil at –20°C. (a) Immediately after quenching; some of the loops, e.g. *A*, contain stacking faults and are Frank sessile dislocations. (b) After being heated slightly; stacking fault in one of the loops has disappeared indicating that the loop is now a unit dislocation. (From WESTMACOTT, BARNES, HULL and SMALLMAN, *Phil. Mag.* **6**, 929, 1961.)

sessile. Thus, considering the negative Frank sessile dislocation in Fig. 5.9, the fault will be removed if the lattice above the fault is sheared so that $C \rightarrow B$, $A \rightarrow C$, $B \rightarrow A$, etc. This is achieved by the movement of a Shockley partial dislocation across the fault. The Shockley partial may have one of three $\frac{1}{6}\langle 112 \rangle$ type vectors lying in the fault plane. It is envisaged that the partial dislocation forms inside the loop and then spreads across the loop removing the fault; at the outside it will react with the Frank partial dislocation to produce a unit slip dislocation according to a reaction of the type

$$\tfrac{1}{6}[11\bar{2}] + \tfrac{1}{3}[111] \;\rightarrow\; \tfrac{1}{2}[110] \qquad (5.7)$$

$$\mathbf{B\alpha} \qquad\quad \mathbf{\alpha A} \qquad\quad \mathbf{BA}$$

Shockley partial    Frank partial    Unit dislocation

Figure 5.10(b) shows the same field as Fig. 5.10(a) after the foil had been in the microscope for some time; the fringe contrast in loop A has disappeared due to a reaction of the type described above and the Burgers vector of the loop has changed from $\frac{1}{3}\langle 111 \rangle \rightarrow \frac{1}{2}\langle 110 \rangle$.

This dislocation reaction will occur only when the stacking fault energy is sufficiently high. The essential problem is whether or not the prevailing conditions in the Frank sessile loop result in the nucleation of a Shockley partial dislocation and allow it to spread across the stacking fault. In the absence of any external shear stress and thermal energy fluctuations the only force tending to create the Shockley partial is that due to the stacking fault in the Frank sessile loop which produces a force $\gamma$ newtons. In section 8.3 it is shown that a shear stress

$$\tau_N \simeq \frac{G}{30} \qquad (5.8)$$

is required to produce a dislocation by homogeneous nucleation. It follows that for a loop with stacking fault energy $\gamma$ there will be spontaneous removal of the fault providing

$$\gamma > \frac{Gb}{30}, \qquad (5.9)$$

where $b$ is the strength of the Burgers vector of the Shockley partial dislocation. Taking $G = 30 \, \text{GN m}^{-2}$ ($3 \times 10^{11}$ dynes cm$^{-2}$) and $\mathbf{b} = \frac{1}{6}[11\bar{2}] = 0.15$ nm gives a minimum stacking fault energy for the removal of the fault $\gamma = 150 \, \text{mJ m}^{-2}$ (ergs cm$^{-2}$), and, therefore, loops formed in all metals with a higher stacking fault energy than this will always consist of unit dislocations without a fault.

This approach sets an upper limit to $\gamma$ for removal of the fault and neglects the effects of thermal vibrations and external stresses on the nucleation of the Shockley partial. A lower limit to $\gamma$ is set by the condition that the energy of the Frank sessile loop with its associated stacking fault is greater than the energy of the unit dislocation loop, i.e. there is a reduction in energy when the stacking fault is removed from the loop. For a circular loop in a face-centred cubic metal the elastic strain energy is given approximately by

$$E = 2\pi P \frac{G}{4\pi} \ln\left(\frac{R}{r_0}\right) \left[\frac{b_1^2}{(1-\nu)} + \frac{1}{2}\left(b_2^2 + \frac{b_2^2}{(1-\nu)}\right)\right] \quad (5.10)$$

where $\mathbf{P}$ is the radius of the loop, $b_1$ and $b_2$ are the strengths of the components of the Burgers vector of the loop perpendicular and parallel to the plane of the loop. The strain field due to the dislocations on opposite sides of the loop will cancel out at distance $\approx P$ away from the loop $R \approx P$. Therefore

$$E = \frac{PG}{4} \left[b_2^2 + \frac{1}{(1-\nu)} (b_2^2 + 2b_1^2)\right] \ln\left(\frac{R}{r_0}\right). \quad (5.11)$$

For a Frank sessile loop lying in a $\{111\}$ plane $\mathbf{b} = \frac{1}{3}\langle 111 \rangle$, $b_1^2 = a^2/3$ and $b_2^2 = 0$, and for a unit dislocation loop, $\mathbf{b} = \frac{1}{2}\langle 110 \rangle$, $b_1^2 = a^2/3$ and $b_2^2 = a^2/6$. Thus, the difference in energy between the loop containing the fault and the loop without the fault is

$$\Delta E = \pi P^2 \gamma - \frac{PGa^2}{24} \left(\frac{2-\nu}{1-\nu}\right) \ln\left(\frac{R}{r_0}\right). \quad (5.12)$$

Therefore, the reaction will be energetically favourable if

$$\gamma > \frac{Ga^2}{24\pi P} \left(\frac{2-\nu}{1-\nu}\right) \ln\left(\frac{R}{r_0}\right). \quad (5.13)$$

Thus the lower limit to the value of $\gamma$ for removal of a fault depends on the size of the loop. Taking $a = 0.35$ nm, $P| = 10$ nm $r_0 = 0.5$ nm, and $v = 0.33$ the critical stacking fault energy is about 36 mJ m$^{-2}$. Since $P| = 10$ nm is close to the minimum size for resolving loops in the electron microscope it is not surprising that stacking fault fringes are rarely observed in metals with $\gamma \gtrsim 40$ mJ m$^{-2}$. As loops containing faults grow by, for example, continual vacancy condensation they will become increasingly less stable. However, the energy required to form a Shockley partial is independent of $P$ and is too large to be created by thermal activation so that it does not follow necessarily that the stable configuration will be achieved. However, the observation in Fig. 5.10 shows that removal of a fault can occur and this is probably due to the presence of local shear stresses in the foil.

### 5.6 Lomer–Cottrell Sessile Dislocation

Strain hardening in metals can be attributed to the progressive introduction during straining of barriers to the free movement of dislocations. The exact nature of these "barriers" is still a matter for conjecture; one specific barrier proposed and observed in face-centred cubic metals is the *Lomer–Cottrell sessile dislocation*. It can be formed in the following way. Consider two unit dislocations $\frac{1}{2}[\bar{1}10]$ and $\frac{1}{2}[101]$ lying in different $\{111\}$ planes and both parallel to the line of intersection of the $\{111\}$ planes (Fig. 5.11). Normally these dislocations will be dissociated and produce extended dislocations which define the $\{111\}$ planes (Fig. 5.11(b)). Under suitable external conditions it is energetically possible for the two leading partial dislocations to interact with each other (Fig. 5.11(c)) according to a reaction of the type

$$\tfrac{1}{6}[\bar{1}2\bar{1}] + \tfrac{1}{6}[1\bar{1}2] \rightarrow \tfrac{1}{6}[011]. \tag{5.14}$$

Applyng the Burgers vector squared criterion there is a reduction in energy from

$$a^2(\tfrac{1}{36} + \tfrac{4}{36} + \tfrac{1}{36}) + a^2(\tfrac{1}{36} + \tfrac{1}{36} + \tfrac{4}{36}) \rightarrow a^2(0 + \tfrac{1}{36} + \tfrac{1}{36}). \tag{5.15}$$

The new dislocation $\frac{1}{6}$[011] lies parallel to the line of intersection of the slip planes and has a pure edge character. The configuration consisting of a wedge-shaped stacking fault ribbon lying in the [0$\bar{1}$1] direction bounded by two partial dislocation, and containing in the edge of the wedge a partial edge dislocation, is a *Lomer-Cottrell dislocation*. The dislocation is *sessile* because the Burgers vector of the dislocation does not lie in either of the planes of its stacking faults (111) and ($\bar{1}$11).

Using Thompson's notation the reactions leading to the Lomer-Cottrell dislocations are as follows:

The unit dislocations **DA** ($\beta$) and **BD** ($\alpha$) dissociate in the $\beta$ and $\alpha$ planes respectively, to form Shockley partial dislocations.

$$\mathbf{DA}(\beta) \to \mathbf{D\beta} \to \mathbf{\beta A}, \qquad (5.16)$$
$$\mathbf{BD}(\alpha) \to \mathbf{B\alpha} + \mathbf{\alpha D}.$$

Two Shockley partials react to form the new partial dislocation

$$\mathbf{\alpha D} + \mathbf{D\beta} \to \mathbf{\alpha\beta} \qquad \text{(Lomer-Cottrell dislocation)} \qquad (5.17)$$

The dislocation configuration produced contains three partial dislocations $\mathbf{\beta A}$, $\mathbf{B\alpha}$, and $\mathbf{\alpha\beta}$. The same configuration could conceivably be formed by the dissociation of a unit dislocation **BA** according to reaction

$$\mathbf{BA} \to \mathbf{B\alpha} + \mathbf{\alpha\beta} + \mathbf{\beta A} \qquad (5.18)$$

since there is a reduction in energy, according to the Burgers vector squared criterion.

Lomer–Cottrell dislocations lie in six possible orientations. The line of the dislocations can be represented by the edges of the Thompson tetrahedron and their Burgers vector by the lines joining the centres of the faces of the tetrahedron, $\alpha\beta$, $\beta\alpha$, $\gamma\alpha$, $\beta\alpha$, $\gamma\beta$ and $\alpha\gamma$.

In Fig. 5.11(c) the stacking fault can be considered to bend from one close-packed plane to the other. The dislocation formed at the intersection is called a *stair rod dislocation*. The $\alpha\beta$-type dislocations discussed above are particular examples of stair-rod dislocations.

9*

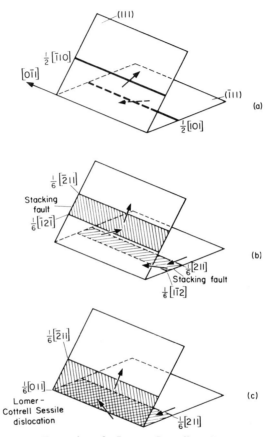

FIG. 5.11. Formation of a Lomer–Cottrell sessile dislocation.

In general stair rod dislocations will form at the intersection of slip planes in which the partials combine, providing the dislocation reaction is energetically favourable (Whelan, 1959).

## 5.7 Tetrahedral Defects

Another dislocation arrangement has been observed in quenched gold by Silcox and Hirsch (1959). This consists of a tetrahedron of stacking faults on {111} planes with $\frac{1}{6}\langle110\rangle$ type stair-rod dislocations along the edges of the tetrahedron. Gold has a relatively low stacking fault energy $\sim 50$ mJ m$^{-2}$ and therefore, according to the criterion in section 5.5, when a platelet of vacancies (produced by quenching from a high temperature) collapses to form a Frank sessile dislocation, the stacking fault will be stable. The Frank sessile may dissociate into a low-energy stair-rod dislocation and a Shockley partial on an intersecting slip plane according to a reaction of the type.

$$\tfrac{1}{3}[111] \rightarrow \tfrac{1}{6}[101]+\tfrac{1}{6}[121], \qquad (5.19)$$

Energy $\propto \qquad\qquad \tfrac{1}{3} \quad \tfrac{1}{18} \quad \tfrac{1}{6}.$

Discounting the energy of the stacking fault there is a reduction in the total energy, and the reaction is energetically favourable. Suppose that the vacancies condense on the {111} plane $\alpha$ in the form of an equilateral triangle with edges parallel to $\langle110\rangle$ directions $BC$, $CD$, $DB$ (Fig. 5.12). The Frank sessile $\alpha A$ can dissociate to produce three Shockley

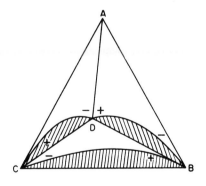

FIG. 5.12. Formation of a tetrahedral defect. This is a physical picture of the reaction (5.20) showing partials $\beta A$, $\gamma A$ and $\delta A$ bowing out in the slip planes $ACD$, $ADB$ and $ABC$ respectively. The relative signs of the dislocations near the nodes are indicated. (From SILCOX and HIRSCH, *Phil. Mag.* **4**, 72, 1959.)

dislocations by reactions of the type (5.19), namely:

$$\alpha A \rightarrow \alpha \beta + \beta A,$$
$$\alpha A \rightarrow \alpha \gamma + \gamma A,$$
$$\alpha A \rightarrow \alpha \delta + \delta A. \qquad (5.20)$$

The partial dislocations $\beta A$, $\alpha A$ and $\gamma A$ will be repelled by the stair rod dislocations $\alpha \beta$, $\alpha \gamma$ and $\alpha \delta$ respectively and will bow out in their slip planes. Taking account of dislocation sign, it is found that the partials attract each other in pairs to form another set of stair rods along *DA*, *BA* and *CA* (Fig. 5.12) according to the reactions

$$\beta A + A\gamma \rightarrow \beta \gamma,$$
$$\gamma A + A\delta \rightarrow \gamma \delta,$$
$$\delta A + A\beta \rightarrow \delta \beta. \qquad (5.21)$$

In vector notation the reactions are of the type (5.14).

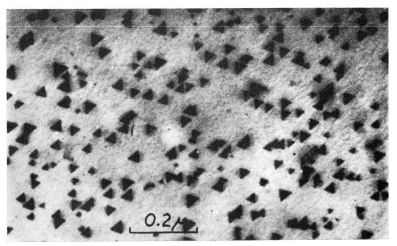

FIG. 5.13. Transmission electron micrograph of tetrahedral defects in quenched gold. The shape of the tetrahedra viewed in transmission depends on their orientation with respect to the plane of the foil, (110) foil orientation. (From COTTRELL, *Phil. Mag.* **6**, 1351, 1961.)

The shape of these tetrahedra observed in thin foils by transmission microscopy depends on the orientation of the tetrahedra with respect to the plane of the foil. An example is shown in Fig. 5.13. The complex contrast patterns inside the faults arise from overlapping stacking faults in different faces of the tetrahedron. The increase in energy due to the formation of stacking faults places a limit on the size of the fault that can be formed. The tetrahedron will form only when the total energy (self-energy of the dislocations and energy of stacking faults) in the tetrahedron is less than the energy of the Frank sessile loop from which it forms.

*Further Reading*

COTTRELL, A. H. (1953) *Dislocations and Plastic Flow in Crystals*, Oxford University Press.

HOWIE, A. (1961) "Quantitative experimental study of dislocations and stacking faults by transmission electron microscopy", *Metallurgical Reviews*, **6**, 467.

KELLY, A. and GROVES, G. W. (1970) *Crystallography and Crystal Defects*, Longmans.

READ, W. T. (1953) *Dislocations in Crystals*, McGraw-Hill, New York.

SEEGER, A. (1957) "Glide and work hardening in face-centred cubic metals", *Dislocations and Mechanical Properties of Crystals*, p. 243, Wiley, New York.

SILCOX, J. and HIRSCH, P. B. (1959) "Direct observations of defects in quenched gold", *Phil. Mag.* **4**, 72.

STEEDS, J. W. (1966) "Dislocation arrangements in copper single crystals as a function of strain", *Proc. Roy. Soc.* A **292**, 343.

SWANN, P. R. (1963) "Dislocation arrangements in face-centred cubic metals and alloys", *Electron Microscopy and Strength of Crystals*, p. 131, Interscience, New York.

THOMPSON, N. (1953) "Dislocation nodes in face-centred cubic lattices", *Proc, Phys. Soc.* B, **66**, 481.

WHELAN, M. J. (1959) "Dislocation interactions in face-centred cubic metals", *Proc. Roy. Soc.* A, **249**, 114.

CHAPTER 6

# Dislocations in Other Crystal Structures

## 6.1 Hexagonal Crystals

In close-packed hexagonal metals, e.g. magnesium, zinc and cadmium, the most closely packed plane is the (0001) *basal plane* and the close-packed directions are $\langle 11\bar{2}0 \rangle$. The smallest unit lattice vector is $\frac{1}{3}\langle 11\bar{2}0 \rangle$. Thus slip is most likely to occur on the basal plane in the $\langle 11\bar{2}0 \rangle$ directions by the movement of dislocations with a Burgers vector $\frac{1}{3}\langle 11\bar{2}0 \rangle$. This mode of deformation has been observed in all the close-packed hexagonal metals. A number of other slip systems have also been observed but, in general, they only occur when basal slip is inhibited for one reason or another.

## 6.2 Dislocations in Hexagonal Crystals

A notation, similar to the Thompson tetrahedron used to describe dislocations in face-centred cubic metals, has been devised by Berghezan, Fourdeux and Amelinckx (1961). A bipyramid is used instead of the tetrahedron and is illustrated in Fig. 6.1. The types of dislocation which are likely to be stable, based on the assumption that the energy of a dislocation is proportional to the square of its Burgers vector, have been listed by Frank and Nicholas (1953) and Berghezan, Fourdeux and Amelinckx as follows:

(a) Six perfect dislocations with Burgers vectors in the basal plane

122

along the sides of the triangular base *ABC* of the pyramid. They are **AB, BC, CA, BA, CB** and **AC**.

(b) Two perfect dislocations perpendicular to the basal plane, represented by the vectors **ST** and **TS**.

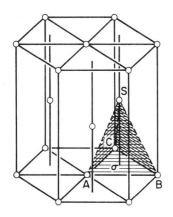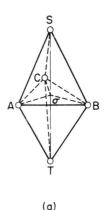

(a)

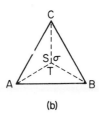

(b)

FIG. 6.1. Burgers vectors in the hexagonal close-packed lattice. (From BERGHEZAN, FOURDEUX and AMELINCKX, *Acta Metall.* **9**, 464, 1960.)

(c) Twelve perfect dislocations of type $\frac{1}{3}[11\bar{2}3]$, whose Burgers vectors are represented by symbols such as **SA/TB,** which means either the sum of the vectors **ST** and **AB** or, geometrically, a vector equal to twice the join of the midpoints of *SA* and *TB*.

(d) Imperfect dislocations perpendicular to the basal plane, namely, σS, σT, Sσ and Tσ.

(e) Imperfect basal dislocations of the Shockley partial type **Aσ, Bσ, Cσ, σA, σB** and **σC**.

(f) Imperfect dislocations which are a combination of the latter two types given by **AS, BS,** etc. Although these vectors represent a displacement from one atomic site to another the associated dislocations are not perfect. This is because the atoms surrounding the two sites are in different orientations and, therefore, it would be impossible to draw a Burgers circuit through a completely good crystal.

The strength, direction and energy of these dislocations in terms of the normal lattice parameters are given in the table, assuming ideal close-packing (section 1.2). Appropriate adjustments are required when dealing with crystal structures which have non-ideal packing.

TABLE 6.1

*Dislocations in Hexagonal Close-packed Structures*

| Type | **AB** | **ST** | **SA/TB** | **Aσ** | **σS** | **AS** |
|---|---|---|---|---|---|---|
| Direction | $[11\bar{2}0]$ | $[000\bar{1}]$ | $[11\bar{2}3]$ | $[\bar{1}100]$ | $[0001]$ | $[\bar{2}203]$ |
| Magnitude | $a$ | $c$ | $\sqrt{(c^2+a^2)}$ | $a/\sqrt{3}$ | $c/2$ | $\sqrt{\left(\dfrac{a^2}{3}+\dfrac{c^2}{4}\right)}$ |
| Energy $\propto$ | $a^2$ | $c^2 = \frac{8}{3}a^2$ | $\frac{11}{3}a^2$ | $\frac{1}{3}a^2$ | $\frac{2}{3}a^2$ | $a^2$ |

A number of different types of stacking faults are associated with the partial dislocations listed in Table 6.1. These faults will have different energies according to the number of bonds which violate the next nearest neighbour rule. The three types of fault which are important all lie in the basal plane; one is associated with glide and the other two are associated principally with dislocation loops introduced by producing platelets of vacancies or interstitials (cf. Face-centred cubic metals, Chapter 5).

## 6.3 Glide in Hexagonal Crystals

As mentioned above the most common slip system is on the basal plane in a close-packed direction $(0001)$ $[11\bar{2}0]$ (basal glide). This is very similar to the $(111)$ $[1\bar{1}0]$ slip in face-centred cubic metals.

The unit slip dislocation $\frac{1}{3}[11\bar{2}0] = \mathbf{AB}$ can dissociate into two partial dislocations bounding a narrow ribbon of stacking fault:

$$\mathbf{AB} = \mathbf{A\sigma} + \mathbf{\sigma B}. \tag{6.1}$$

The spacing of the partials will be inversely proportional to the stacking fault energy (section 5.3). Recent estimates suggest that $\gamma$ is about 20 mJ m$^{-2}$ for cadmium and zinc and considerably higher for magnesium. The dissociation of unit dislocations in a single crystal platelet containing an **AB** dislocation was studied experimentally by Price (1963). The platelet was strained in such a way that

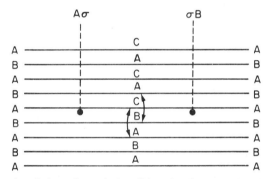

F<small>IG</small>. 6.2. Dissociation of a unit **AB** dislocation into two Shockley partial dislocations separated by a stacking fault.

the force on the total dislocation was zero; i.e. the angle between the Burgers vector of the dislocation and the direction of the applied stress was 90°. However, in this orientation the force produced by this stress on the two partials **Aσ** and **σB** was finite, equal and opposite. At a particular stress determined by the stacking fault energy the partial dislocations moved in opposite directions to infinity (the retarding force due to the surface tension of the stacking fault is independent of distance). The stacking fault sequence produced by basal dissociation of glide dislocations is illustrated in Fig. 6.2. The arrows indicate that there are two violations of the nearest neighbour rule.

Glide will tend to be restricted to the basal plane for two reasons, firstly because the unit dislocation is dissociated in this plane and secondly, because there is no other close-packed plane intersecting the basal plane, as in face-centred cubic metals. Cross slip, therefore, is a difficult process. However, slip on other systems has been observed. The most common is *pyramidal glide* on $(10\bar{1}1)$ $[\bar{1}2\bar{1}0]$ and, in addition, *prismatic glide* has been observed on $(10\bar{1}0)$ $[\bar{1}2\bar{1}0]$. In bulk specimens, in which the dislocations usually lie on basal planes, this can occur by cross slip. This is illustrated in Fig. 6.3. An undissociated screw

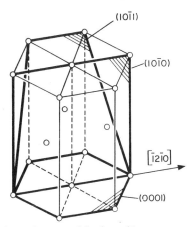

FIG. 6.3. Planes in an hexagonal lattice with a common $[\bar{1}2\bar{1}0]$ direction.

dislocation lying along $[\bar{1}2\bar{1}0]$ which normally glides in the basal plane, can move in either the pyramidal or prismatic planes, providing that glide on the basal plane is restricted either by an obstacle or an unfavourable stress field. Since the onset of cross slip necessitates the constriction of the stacking fault ribbons of the screw dislocation, glide on $(10\bar{1}1)$ and $(10\bar{1}0)$ will be favoured at high temperatures and in metals with a high stacking fault energy. This is in broad agreement with the experimental observations.

In very small platelets, initially free from dislocations, it has been possible to nucleate dislocations at the edges when the platelets are strained in the electron microscope (Price, 1963). By choosing a suitable orientation, glide on the basal planes can be prevented, and it is observed that **AB** dislocations can be nucleated which glide directly on (10$\bar{1}$1). It has also been possible in cadmium and zinc platelets to nucleate **SA/TB** dislocations which have an energy almost four times greater than **AB** dislocations (see Table 6.1). The glide plane was the (11$\bar{2}$2) second-order pyramidal plane and frequent cross slip was observed even at low temperatures. Although these dislocations were formed and moved under very severe and unusual stress conditions, they illustrate that high-energy dislocations will form when formation of low-energy dislocations is restricted. The (11$\bar{2}$2) [$\bar{1}\bar{1}$23] system has been indentified in bulk crystals.

## 6.4 Vacancy and Interstitial Loops
## in Hexagonal Crystals

As in face-centred cubic metals, vacancies, which may be formed by energetic particle irradiation, plastic deformation or quenching, tend to precipitate as platelets on close-packed planes. However, when this occurs in close-packed hexagonal metals (Fig. 6.4(a)) it results in two similar layers coming into contact (Fig. 6.4(b)). This is a very unfavourable situation which can be avoided by one of two mechanisms:

(i) by changing the stacking of one layer into a C position (Fig. 6.4(c)),

(ii) by having the loop swept by a partial dislocation that changes the stacking sequence above the loop according to a rule of the type $A \to B \to C \to A$ (Fig. 6.4(d)).

In (i) (Fig. 6.4(c)), the Burgers vector of the dislocation loop is of the type **σS**. The loop contains a high-energy stacking fault because there are three violations of the next-nearest-neighbour rule (as shown by the arrows). In (ii) (Fig. 6.4(d)), the Burgers vector of the loop is of the type **AS** and the associated stacking fault is a low-energy fault because there is only one violation of the next-nearest-neighbour rule. Since there is a large decrease in stacking fault energy from (i) to (ii) it is possible that (i) is unstable with respect to (ii). The change will be produced if a partial dislocation **Aσ** is nucleated which sweeps across the loop (see section 5.5.). The dislocation reaction

$$\mathbf{A\sigma + \sigma S = AS} \qquad (6.2)$$

will occur so producing the low-energy fault (ii). A simple calculation

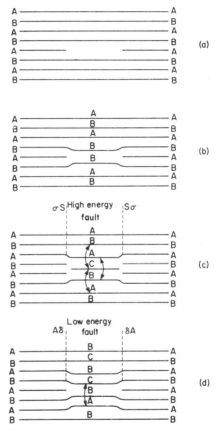

FIG. 6.4. Formation of prismatic dislocation loops as a result of the precipitation of one layer of vacancies. (a) Disc-shaped cavity. (b) Collapse of the disc bringing two *B* layers together. (c) Formation of a high-energy stacking fault. (d) Formation of a low-energy stacking fault. The actual sequence of planes formed will depend on the plane in which the vacancies form, i.e. *A* or *B*. It is possible to have loops of the same form with different Burgers vectors lying on adjacent planes. (After BERGHEZAN, FOURDEUX and AMELINCKX, *Acta Metall.* **9**, 464, 1961.)

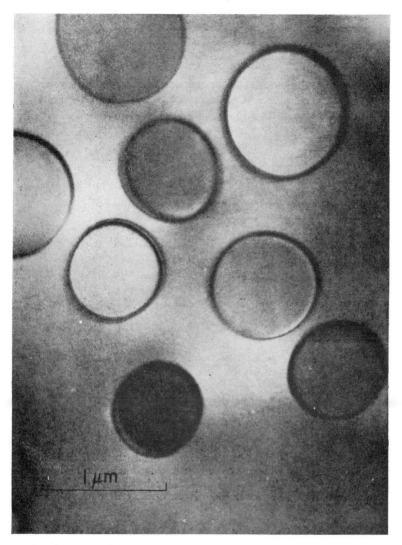

FIG. 6.5. Transmission electron micrograph of dislocation loops of the **SA** type produced in a cadmium crystal by bombardment with energetic ions. The loops enclose low-energy stacking faults; the normal fringe contrast does not occur because the plane of the loops is parallel to the plane of the foil specimen. (From PRICE, *Phys. Rev. Letters*, **6**, 615, 1961.)

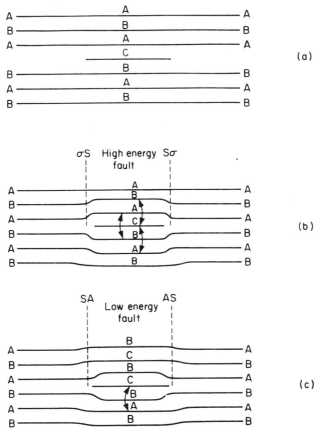

Fig. 6.6. (a) Precipitation of a layer of interstitials. (b) Prismatic loop resulting from the layer of interstitials: the loop contains a high-energy stacking fault. (c) Prismatic loop containing low-energy stacking fault. (After Berghezan, Fourdeux and Amelinckx, *Acta Metall.* **9**, 464, 1961.)

shows that there is a critical size of loop above which this sequence is energetically favourable.

It is also possible to produce loops enclosing stacking faults by the precipitation of interstitial atoms into platelets. Thus, in Fig. 6.6, the insertion of a *C* layer results in the formation of a loop of dislocation with Burgers vector **So** and a high-energy stacking fault with three violations of the next-nearest-neighbour rule. This high-energy fault can again be changed to a low-energy fault by having the loop swept by a partial of the type **σA** which will change the Burgers vector of the loop to **SA** (Fig. 6.6).

The dislocation loops formed from vacancy or interstitial platelets are free to climb in the same way as the loops in face-centred cubic metals and so will expand or contract depending on the sign of the dislocation and the prevailing conditions (section 3.6).

Finally it should be mentioned that not all the possible situations have been described. More complex loops are possible, when for example, two layers of vacancies or interstitials are introduced.

### 6.5 Dislocations in Body-centred Cubic Crystals

In body-centred cubic metals (e.g. iron, molybdenum, tantalum, vanadium, chromium, tungsten, niobium, sodium and potassium) *slip* occurs in close-packed $\langle 111 \rangle$ directions. The shortest lattice vector extends from a cube corner to the atom at the centre of the unit cell. Thus the Burgers vector of the unit slip dislocation is of the type $\frac{1}{2}\langle 111 \rangle$. The slip plane has variously been reported as $\{110\}$, $\{112\}$ and $\{123\}$. Each of these planes contain $\langle 111 \rangle$ slip directions and it is particularly significant that three $\{110\}$, three $\{112\}$ and six $\{123\}$ planes intersect along the same $\langle 111 \rangle$ direction. Thus, if cross slip is easy it is possible for screw dislocations to move in a haphazard way on different $\{110\}$ planes or combinations of $\{110\}$ and $\{112\}$ planes, etc., favoured by the applied stress. For this reason slip lines are often wavy and ill-defined. It has been found that the apparent slip plane varies with composition, temperature and strain rate. Thus, when pure iron is deformed at room temperature the slip plane appears to be close to the maximum resolved shear stress plane irrespective of the position of the crystallographic orientation, whereas when it is deformed at low temperatures, or alloyed with silicon, slip tends to be restricted to a specific $\{110\}$ plane.

An interesting feature in body-centred cubic metals which has been studied extensively in recent years is the asymmetry of slip. It is found, for example, that the slip plane of a single crystal deformed in uniaxial compression may be different from the slip plane which operates in tension for the same crystal orientation. In other words, the shear stress to move a dislocation lying in a slip plane in one direction is not the same as the shear stress required to move it in the opposite

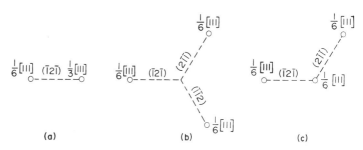

FIG. 6.7. Dissociation of screw dislocations an {112} planes: (a) glissile split-tung, (b) unstable sessile splitting, (c) stable sessile splitting.

direction in the same plane. This observation indicates that the dislocation is not behaving like a perfect unit $\frac{1}{2}\langle 111 \rangle$ dislocation and that it is either dissociated or the atoms at the centre or core of the dislocation have relaxed into a particular asymmetric configuration. The ease of cross slip referred to earlier indicates that the amount of dissociation is small and this is confirmed by the very high stacking-fault energy predicted for most body-centred cubic metals, $\gamma \sim 200$ to $1000\,\mathrm{mJ\,m^{-2}}$. However, a number of dissociations of the $\frac{1}{2}\langle 111 \rangle$ dislocations are geometrically possible and the most important are those which lead to the formation of $\frac{1}{6}\langle 111 \rangle$ dislocations.

The occurrence of {112} $\langle 111 \rangle$ twinning in body-centred cubic metals suggests that dissociation may occur on {112} planes resulting in a {112} stacking fault, Fig. 6.7. Dissociation of the $\frac{1}{2}\langle 111 \rangle$ dislocation in a {112} plane can occur as follows:

$$\frac{1}{2}[111] \rightarrow \frac{1}{3}[111] + \frac{1}{6}[111]. \qquad (6.3)$$

This results in a reduction in elastic strain energy from $\frac{3}{4} \rightarrow \frac{5}{12}$ and is therefore energetically favoured. However, a "twin" stacking fault will form between the two partials and since their Burgers vectors are parallel the partials cannot be separated by a homogeneous shear stress. When the dislocation line is parallel to [111] both dislocations will be screw orientated and can glide on any of the three {112} planes which intersect along [111]. A further possibility then suggests itself; the $\frac{1}{2}$[111] dislocation could dissociate and form a 'tripod' fault with three $\frac{1}{6}$[111] partial dislocations lying in three {112} planes as shown in Fig. 6.7b,

$$\frac{1}{2}[111] \rightarrow \frac{1}{6}[111] + \frac{1}{6}[111] + \frac{1}{6}[111]. \tag{6.4}$$

It has been shown that tripod arrangement is not a stable configuration and that it is more likely for the arrangement of the triple splitting to be as shown in Fig. 6.7c. It will be clear from models of this kind that subsequent movement of dislocations which have dissociated in the way illustrated in Fig. 6.7c or have an asymmetrical core configuration will be dependent on the direction of movement in the slip plane.

Splitting or dissociation of dislocations has also been proposed to occur on {110} planes and the two best known proposals are

$$\frac{1}{2}[111] \rightarrow \frac{1}{8}[110] + \frac{1}{4}[112] + \frac{1}{8}[110] \tag{6.5}$$

which would occur entirely in a ($\bar{1}$10) slip plane and is glissile, and

$$\frac{1}{2}[111] \rightarrow \frac{1}{8}[110] + \frac{1}{8}[101] + \frac{1}{8}[011] + \frac{1}{4}[111] \tag{6.6}$$

which involves a screw dislocation splitting on three {110} planes of the same $\langle 111 \rangle$ zone. This dissociation leads to a sessile dislocation since the dislocation cannot glide unless the dislocation constricts.

Another possible group of unit dislocations in body-centred cubic metals are the $\langle 100 \rangle$ dislocations. They are formed when two $\frac{1}{2}\langle 111 \rangle$ slip dislocations interact as follows:

$$\frac{1}{2}[\bar{1}\bar{1}1] + \frac{1}{2}[111] \rightarrow [001]. \tag{6.7}$$

This reaction results in a reduction of elastic strain energy and the properties of the [001] dislocation formed will depend on whether or not it has an edge, screw or mixed character. In the pure edge orientation the Burgers vector is at right angles to the main cleavage plane in body-centred cubic metals and it has been suggested that the $\langle 100 \rangle$ dislocations are responsible for crack initiation. In the screw orientation the $\langle 100 \rangle$ dislocation could glide on $\{110\}$ planes but this process is not nearly so significant as $\langle 111 \rangle$ slip. Interaction of $\frac{1}{2} \langle 111 \rangle$ dislocations could also result in the formation of $\langle 110 \rangle$ dislocations, viz.

$$\tfrac{1}{2}[\bar{1}11] + \tfrac{1}{2}[111] \rightarrow [011], \qquad (6.8)$$

but the energetics suggest that this is unlikely.

*Deformation twinning* is observed in all the body-centred cubic transition metals when they are deformed at low temperatures. The crystallography is identical for all these metals and twinning occurs on $\{112\} \langle 111 \rangle$ systems. In section 1.2 it was shown that the stacking sequence of $\{112\}$ planes in the body-centred cubic structure is $ABCDEFAB \ldots$ The homogeneous shear required to produce a twin is $1\sqrt{2}$ in a $\langle 111 \rangle$ direction on a $\{112\}$ plane. This shear can be produced by a displacement of $\frac{1}{6}\langle 111 \rangle$ on every successive $\{112\}$ plane and this led to the suggestion that twinning occurs by the movement of $\frac{1}{6}\langle 111 \rangle$ partial dislocations in the way illustrated in Fig. 6.8. The diagram (Fig. 6.8(a)) shows a $(1\bar{1}0)$ section through a body-centred cubic lattice. The $\{112\}$ *twin composition plane* or *twinning plane* is normal to the $(1\bar{1}0)$ plane and its trace is shown on the diagram. When a set of twinning dislocations, lying along $XY$, moves as in Fig. 6.8(b) the volume swept out is twinned. Figure 6.8(c) shows the final twin related structure, the twinning dislocations having crossed the whole crystal. Evidence for twinning dislocations of this type has been observed in a body-centred cubic molybdenum–rhenium alloy which twins profusely when deformed, even at relatively high temperatures. Figure 6.9(b) shows a thin film electron transmission micrograph of a small twin. Each change in the contrast sequence coincides with a partial dislocation as illustrated diagrammatically in Fig. 6.9(c) and the movement of each partial produces a change in the stacking sequence as illustrated in Fig. 6.8.

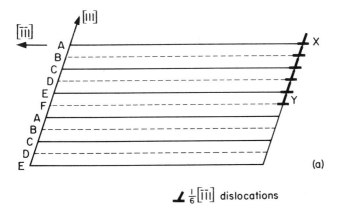

$\swarrow \frac{1}{6}[\bar{1}\bar{1}1]$ dislocations

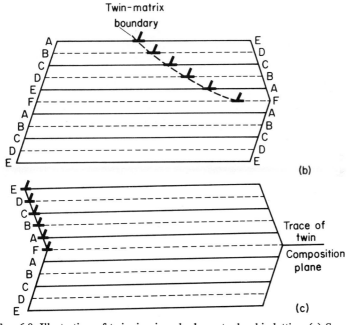

FIG. 6.8. Illustration of twinning in a body-centred cubic lattice. (a) Section parallel to (1$\bar{1}$0) showing the stacking sequence of (112) planes. $X$–$Y$ is a row of $\frac{1}{6}[\bar{1}\bar{1}1]$ twinning dislocations; one dislocation on each (112) plane. (b) The twinning dislocations have moved part way across the crystal to produce a twin orientated region; note the change in stacking sequence. (c) A twinned crystal.

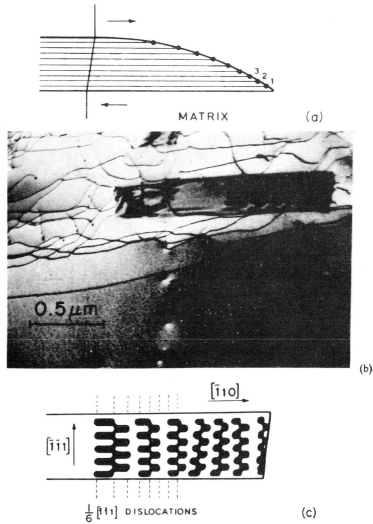

MATRIX (a)

(b)

$[\bar{1}10]$

$[\bar{1}\bar{1}1]$

$\frac{1}{6}[\bar{1}\bar{1}1]$ DISLOCATIONS (c)

FIG. 6.9. Experimental observation of a small deformation twin in a molybdenum 35 per cent rhenium alloy by transmission electron microscopy. (a) Illustration of the shape of the small twin shown in (b); the dislocations are represented by dots. (b) Diffraction contrast produced by twin which lies at an angle of 20° to the plane of the thin foil. (c) Diagrammatic illustration of the diffraction contrast observed in (b). Each change in the fringe sequence is due to a twinning dislocation. (From HULL (1962), *Proc. 5th Int. Conf. Electron Microscopy*, p. B9, Academic Press.)

## 6.6 Dislocations in Other Crystal Structures

Dislocations in more complex lattices obey similar rules to those in face-centred and body-centred cubic and close-packed hexagonal lattices, but are themselves more complex and less easily identified by a simple analysis of the structure. The structures discussed so far have been made up of atoms of one element only (i.e. pure metals). Other factors become important in considering the structure and movement of dislocations in crystals composed of two or more elements. Some of these factors will be illustrated with reference to ionic crystals, super lattices, layer structures and polymer crystals.

DISLOCATIONS IN IONIC CRYSTALS

Non-metallic inorganic crystals consist of cations and anions arranged on a crystal lattice. The simplest structures have cubic symmetry and fall into two groups referred to as the sodium chloride (NaCl) type structure and the caesium chloride (CsCl) type structure. The NaCl structure (Fig. 1.13) may be considered as two interpenetrating face-centred cubic lattices of the two types of atom, with the corner of one located at the point $\frac{1}{2}$, 0, 0 of the other. The CsCl structure consists of two interpenetrating simple cubic lattices of the two types of atom with the corner of one located at the point $\frac{1}{2}, \frac{1}{2}, \frac{1}{2}$ of the other. A number of materials, e.g. MgO, LiF, and AgCl, have the NaCl structure and have been studied in great detail. Although the sodium and chlorine atoms actually exist in the lattice as cations and anions respectively they occur in equal numbers and the net charge of the crystal is zero. If the atoms were all the same the lattice would be simple cubic and the shortest lattice vector and hence the predicted slip direction would be along $\langle 100 \rangle$ directions. The slip plane would be (010). However, if this occurred in the NaCl lattice the sodium ions in one layer would move close to sodium ions in the adjacent layers, and similarly with the chlorine ions. This is very unfavourable energetically and does not occur. The only low index directions that lie parallel to rows of ions of the same charge sign are $\langle 110 \rangle$. Glide can occur in these directions without juxtaposing ions of the same sign. Also the smallest crystallographic repeat distance lies in the $\langle 110 \rangle$ direction. Thus, the predicted slip dislocation is $\frac{1}{2}\langle 110 \rangle$ and this is in agreement with experimental observations of slip in these crystals. The principal slip plane is of the $\{110\}$ type but there are a few observations of slip on $\{100\}$ particularly at high temperatures. An additional effect is that as the temperature increases the ionic nature of the bonding decreases and hence the ionic restrictions to glide are relaxed. *Cross slip* of screw dislocations can occur only by slip on a plane other than a $\{110\}$ plane since only one $\langle 110 \rangle$ direction is contained in a given $\{110\}$ plane.

Figure 6.10 shows a diagrammatic representation of a pure edge dislocation with a $\frac{1}{2}[110]$ Burgers vector and $(1\bar{1}0)$ slip plane. The chlorine ions are represented by $-$ and the sodium ions by $+$. The ions in the planes immediately above and below the one illustrated are in exactly the same position, but of opposite sign. Thus, the edge dislocation contains two extra half planes of the $\{110\}$ type. The two half planes are necessary to maintain the charge balance. Separation of the half planes, as in the dissociation of a $\frac{1}{2}\langle 110 \rangle$ dislocation in a face-centred metal, is very unlikely because (a) separation of the planes would break the charge balance, (b) there would be no reduction in the strain energy, and (c) the stacking fault that would be produced would have a large energy because of the change in the charge distribution.

Figure 6.10 also serves to illustrate that there is an effective charge associated with the emergence point of a $\frac{1}{2}[1\bar{1}0]$ dislocation in the (001) plane. This can be either positive or negative. There is no charge when the emergence point is in the (110) plane. Charges are associated with jogs on dislocation lines as illustrated in Fig. 6.11. Part of the extra half planes end inside the crystal and produce jogs on the dislocation. There is one negative charge in excess which is divided between the two end points of the row, i.e. between the two jogs. Thus, the effective charge of the jog is $e/2$. Addition of a positive ion to the row displaces the jog sideways and inverts the sign of the effective charge at the jog.

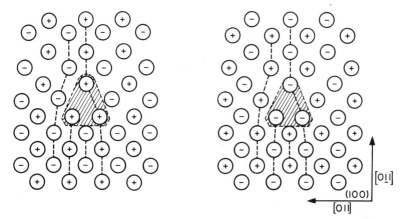

FIG. 6.10. Edge dislocation in NaCl structure. The glide plane is ($1\bar{1}0$) and the Burgers vector $\frac{1}{2}[110]$. The shaded region illustrates that there is an effective charge associated with the emergence site of the dislocation in the (001) plane of the diagram. (From AMELINCKX, Supplement Vol. 7, Series X, *Nuovo Cimento*, p. 569, 1958.)

DISLOCATIONS IN SUPERLATTICES

In many solid solutions of one element in another the different species of atoms are arranged at random on the atomic positions of the lattice. At a composition *AB*, for example, any given lattice point is occupied indifferently by either *A* or *B* atoms. There are some solid solutions, however, in which a specific distribution of the atom species can be induced. Atoms of one kind segregate more or less completely on one set of atomic positions, leaving atoms of the other kind to the remaining positions. The resulting arrangement can be described as a lattice of *A* atoms interpenetrating a lattice of *B* atoms. A random solid solution is changed to an *ordered solid solution* with a *superlattice*. Many possibilities exist in metal and non-metallic alloys; as an example, the superlattice produced in an alloy of composition $AB_3$ will be considered (e.g. $Cu_3Au$ and $Ni_3Mn$). The superlattice of such alloys is illustrated in Fig. 6.12. In the disordered state this is a face-centred cubic lattice and the dislocation behaviour will be similar to that described in Chapter 5. However, in an ordered lattice the posi-

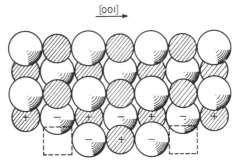

FIG. 6.11. Extra half planes of the edge dislocation in Fig. 6.10 with a jog at each end denoted by the squares. (From AMELINCKX, Supplement Vol. 7, Series X, *Nuovo Cimento*, p. 569, 1958.)

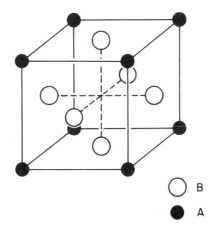

FIG. 6.12. Unit cell of an $AB_3$ superlattice.

tions of the individual atoms become important and this is best demonstrated by considering the simple slip process. The arrangement of atoms in the (111) planes of the ordered lattice is illustrated in Fig. 6.13. A slip vector $\frac{1}{2}[\bar{1}10]$ (unit dislocation in a pure metal) displaces the atoms in the top layer from position $X$ to position $Y$). This produces a change in the local arrangement of the atoms on the (111) slip plane (i.e. an *antiphase domain boundary*, *A.P.B.*). This boundary has a characteristic energy depending on the degree of order

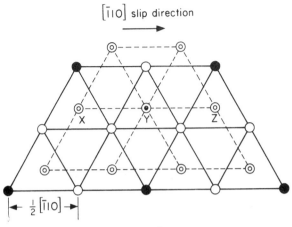

FIG. 6.13. Arrangement of atoms in two adjacent (111) planes in an $AB_3$ superlattice.

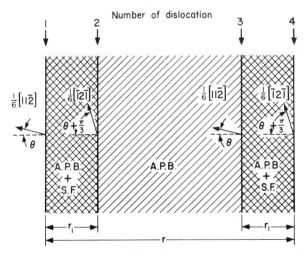

FIG. 6.14. A [01$\bar{1}$] superlattice dislocation in an $AB_3$ superlattice. (From MARCINKOWSKI, BROWN and FISHER, *Acta Met.* **9**, 129, 1961.)

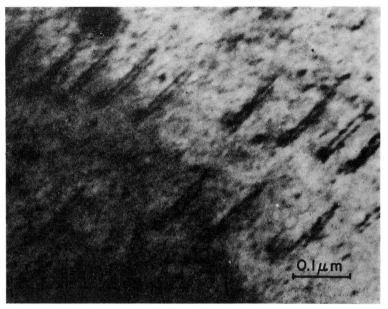

FIG. 6.15. Electron transmission micrograph of a superlattice dislocation in fully ordered Cu₃Au. (From MARCINKOWSKI, BROWN and FISHER, *Acta Met.* **9**, 129, 1961.)

in the lattice. Figure 6.13 shows that the disorder produced by the slip process can be removed by a second $\frac{1}{2}[\bar{1}10]$ dislocation which restores the original atomic arrangement. The top layer is moved from position $Y$ to position $Z$. Thus, the perfect dislocation in the ordered lattice, referred to as a *superlattice dislocation*, consists of two $\frac{1}{2}[\bar{1}10]$ ordinary dislocations joined by an antiphase domain boundary. This is similar to an extended dislocation consisting of two partial dislocations joined by a stacking fault. In the example considered the $\frac{1}{2}[\bar{1}10]$ dislocations themselves will be dissociated into Shockley partials so that the super-lattice dislocation will consist of two extended dislocations connected by an antiphase domain boundary as illustrated in Fig. 6.14. The actual equilibrium separation between the four partials will depend upon the energy of the stacking fault and the energy of the antiphase domain boundary which in turn will depend on the degree of order.

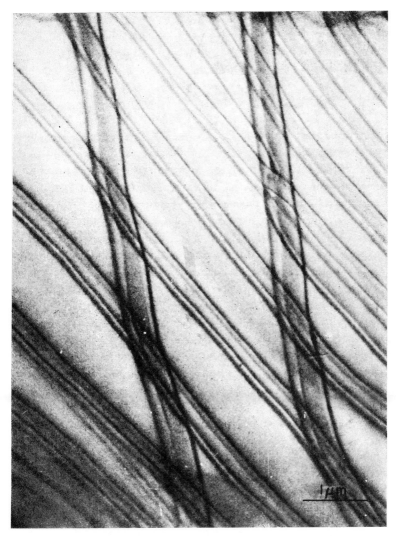

FIG. 6.16. Electron transmission micrograph of dislocation ribbons in talc. (From AMELINCKX and DELAVIGNETTE (1962), *Direct Observation of Imperfections in Crystals*, p. 295, Interscience.)

Figure 6.15 shows an electron transmission micrograph of superlattice dislocations in fully ordered $Cu_3Au$. Each dislocation is represented by two $\frac{1}{2}[110]$ dislocations. The spacing of the partials is too small to be resolved.

### DISLOCATIONS IN LAYER STRUCTURES

There is a large group of materials which have a pronounced layer-type structure which can arise in two ways. Firstly, when the binding forces between atoms in the layers are much stronger than the binding forces between atoms in adjacent layer, as, for example, in graphite. Secondly, when the arrangement of the atoms in complex molecular structures results in the formation of two-dimensional sheets of molecules as, for example, in talc and mica. There are a number of important consequences of the *layer structure*. Slip occurs readily in planes parallel to the layers and is almost impossible in non-layer planes and, therefore, the dislocation arrangements and Burgers vectors are confined mainly to the layer planes. The weak binding between layers results in a low stacking fault energy and hence unit dislocations are widely dissociated into partial dislocations. Figure 6.16 shows an example of dislocations in talc. In this material the unit dislocations dissociate into four component partial dislocations. The dislocations appear as ribbons lying in the layer planes, and in some circumstances the electron diffraction conditions allow all four partials to be observed.

Many studies have been made of crystals with layer structures. They are particularly convenient to study experimentally because uniformly thick specimens for transmission electron microscopy can be obtained simply by cleavage along the layer planes.

### DISLOCATIONS IN POLYMER CRYSTALS

It is now possible to produce single crystals of many polymers, such as polyethylene, and it is also known that bulk semi-crystalline polymers consist of blocks of perfectly crystalline material surrounded by amorphous material. The shape of the crystal blocks or lamellae is illustrated in

Fig. 6.17. These lamellae are very small and typically in high molecular weight polymers the thickness of the blocks is in the range 10 to 100 nm. The polymer chains are usually normal to the plane of the sheet. Figure 6.17 illustrates two other important features of polymer crystals: firstly, the strong covalent bonds of the polymer "backbone" are all aligned parallel to each other, and secondly, because the length of the polymer chain is greater than the thickness of the crystal,

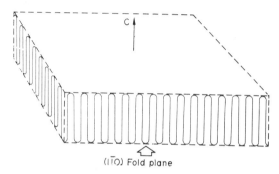

($1\bar{1}0$) Fold plane

Fig. 6.17. Schematic representation of a polymer single crystal showing the nature of the fold structure.

the chains fold over back into the crystal. The fold structure and geometry play an important role in the deformation of polymer crystals.

Many kinds of defect can occur in this type of crystal and a number of different dislocation configurations have been proposed. The weak bonding between molecules means that deformation occurs most readily by sliding parallel to the $c$-axis so that dislocations with Burgers vectors $\langle 00c \rangle$ which glide in (100), (010) and (110) are likely to be preferred. The fold structure introduces a constraint on this kind of intermolecular slip and slip in planes containing the fold will be more pronounced than others.

## Further Reading

### HEXAGONAL CRYSTALS

BERGHEZAN, A., FOURDEUX, A. and AMELINCKX, S. (1961) "Dislocations and stacking faults in a hexagonal metal: zinc", *Acta Metall.* **9**, 464.

FRANK, F. C. and NICHOLAS, J. F. (1953) "Stable dislocations in the common crystal lattices", *Phil. Mag.* **44**, 1213.

PARTRIDGE, P. G. (1968) "Crystallography and defomation modes of hexagonal close-packed metals", *Metals and Materials.*

PRICE, P. B. (1961) "Direct observation of ion damage in cadmium", *Phys. Rev. Letters*, **6**, 615.

PRICE, P. B. (1963) "Observations of glide, climb and twinning in hexagonal metal crystals", *Electron Microscopy and Strength of Crystals*, p. 41, Interscience, New York.

### BODY-CENTRED CUBIC CRYSTALS AND TWINNING

"Deformation of crystalline solids" (1966) Conference proceedings, *Can. J. Phys.*, Vol. **45**, (many important papers).

CARRINGTON, W., HALE, K. F. and McLEAN, D. (1960) "Arrangement of dislocations in iron, *Proc. Roy. Soc.* A, **259**, 203.

DINGLEY, D. J. and HALE, K. F. (1966) "Burgers vectors of dislocations in deformed iron and iron alloys", *Proc. Roy. Soc.* A, **295**, 55.

HULL, D. (1963) "Growth of twins and associated dislocation phenomena", *Twinning*, p. 121, Wiley.

KEH, A. S. and WEISSMANN, S. (1963) "Deformation sub-structure in body-centred cubic metals", *Electron Microscopy and Strength of Crystals*, p. 231, Interscience, New York.

SLEESWYK, A. W. (1962) "Emissary dislocations: theory and experiments on the propagation of deformation in α-iron", *Acta Metall.* **10**, 705.

SLEESWYK, A. W. (1963) "Screw dislocations and the nucleation of twins", *Phil. Mag.* **8**, 1467.

### OTHER CRYSTAL STRUCTURES

ALEXANDER, H. and HAASEN, P. (1972) "Dislocations in non-metals", *Ann. Rev. Mat. Sci.* **2**, 291.

AMELINCKX, S. (1958) "Dislocations in ionic crystals", Supplement to Vol. 7, Series X, *Nuovo Cimento*, p. 569.

AMELINCKX, S. and DELAVIGNETTE, P. (1962) "Dislocations in layer structures", *Direct Observation of Lattice Imperfections*, p. 295, Interscience, New York.

GEIL, P. H. (1963) *Polymer Single Crystals*, Wiley.

GILMAN, J. J. and JOHNSTON, W. G. (1962) "Dislocations in lithium fluoride", *Solid State Physics*, **13**, 147.

MARCINKOWSKI, M. J., BROWN, N. and FISHER, R. M. (1961) "Dislocation configurations in $Cu_3Au$ and AuCu type superlattices", *Acta Metall.* **9**, 129.

MARCINKOWSKI, M. J. (1963) "Theory and direct observation of antiphase boundaries and dislocations in superlattices", *Electron Microscopy and Strength of Crystals*, p. 333, Interscience, New York.

PETERMANN, J. and GLEITER, H. (1972) "Direct observation of dislocations in polyethylene crystals", *Phil. Mag.* **25**, 813.

PREDECKI, P. and STATTON. W. O. (1967) "A dislocation mechanism for deformation in polyethylene", *J. Appl. Phys.* **38**, 4140.

THOMAS, J. M. (1970) "The chemistry of deformed and imperfect crystals", *Endeavour*, **29**, 149.

CHAPTER 7

# Jogs and the Intersection
# of Dislocations

## 7.1 Introduction

It has been shown that dislocations glide freely in certain planes under the action of an applied shear stress. Since even well-annealed crystals contain a network of dislocations it follows that every slip plane will be threaded by dislocations and a dislocation moving in the slip plane will have to intersect the dislocations crossing the slip plane. The latter are called *"forest dislocations"*. As plastic deformation proceeds slip occurs on other slip systems and the slip plane of one system intersects slip planes of the other systems, thus increasing the number of forest dislocations. The ease with which slip occurs depends, to a large degree, on the way the gliding dislocations overcome the barriers provided by the forest dislocations. Since the dislocation density in a crystal increases with increasing strain, the intersection processes affect the rate at which the crystal hardens as it is strained. The elementary features of the intersection process are best understood by considering the geometry of the intersection of straight dislocations moving on orthogonal slip planes.

## 7.2 Intersection of Dislocations

The intersection of two edge dislocations with Burgers vectors at right angles to each other is illustrated in Fig. 7.1. An edge dislocation $XY$ with Burgers vector $\mathbf{b}_1$ is gliding in plane $P_{XY}$. It cuts through

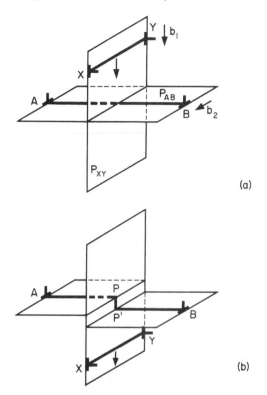

(a)

(b)

FIG. 7.1. Intersection of edge dislocations with Burgers vectors at right angles to each other. (a) A dislocation *XY* moving on its slip plane $P_{XY}$ is about to cut the dislocation *AB* lying in plane $P_{AB}$. (b) *XY* has cut through *AB* and produced a jog *PP′* in *AB*. The formation of the jog can be envisaged by considering the displacement of plane $P_{AB}$ produced by dislocation *XY*. (From READ (1953), *Dislocations in Crystals*, McGraw-Hill.)

dislocation *AB* with Burgers vector $\mathbf{b}_2$ lying in plane $P_{AB}$. The intersection results in a jog *PP′* (see section 3.6) in dislocation *AB* which is parallel to the Burgers vector $\mathbf{b}_1$ of the dislocation *XY*. Since the jog is still part of the dislocation *AB* it has a Burgers vector $\mathbf{b}_2$, but the length of the jog is equal to the length of the Burgers vector $\mathbf{b}_1$. The Burgers vector of dislocation *AB* is parallel to *XY* and no jog will be formed in the dislocation *XY*; the additional strain is relieved

11*

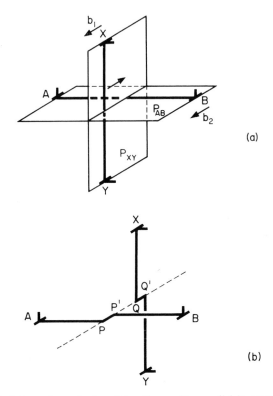

(a)

(b)

Fig. 7.2. Intersection of edge dislocations with parallel Burgers vectors. (a) Before intersection. (b) After intersection.

by glide along the dislocation line. The overall length of the dislocation **AB** is increased by $b_1$. Since the energy per unit length of dislocation is $\alpha G b^2$ where $\alpha \approx 1$ (equation (4.12)) the energy of the jog is $\alpha G b^3$, neglecting the effect of elastic interaction with adjacent dislocations. However, a jog in an undissociated dislocation is a short length of dislocation with practically no long-range elastic energy and $\alpha \ll 1$. The energy is determined, then, by the core energy of the dislocation (section 4.4). A value of $\alpha = 0.2$ will be used.

The intersection of two orthogonal edge dislocations with parallel Burgers vectors is illustrated in Fig. 7.2. Jogs are formed on both dislocations. The length of the jog in $QQ'$ is equal to $b_2$ and the length of the jog in $PP'$ is equal to $b_1$. The increase in energy as a result of the intersection is twice that for the example above.

The intersections of a screw dislocation with an edge dislocation, and a screw dislocation, are illustrated in Figs. 7.3 and 7.4 respectively. The sign of the screw dislocations are represented by the arrows. For the examples given all the screw dislocations are right-handed, according to the definition given in section 1.4. Jogs are produced on all the dislocations after intersection.

The length, or "height", of all the jogs described is equal to the Burgers vector of the intersecting dislocation or, in other words, to the spacing between atom planes. These are referred to as *elementary jogs*.

## 7.3 Movement of Dislocations Containing Elementary Jogs

Consider the jog formed on the edge dislocation $AB$ in Fig. 7.1; the Burgers vector is normal to $PP'$ and it is therefore an *edge dislocation*. The slip plane defined by dislocation $AB$ has a step in it, but the Burgers vector is at all times in the slip plane. Thus, the jog will glide along with the dislocation. The jogs formed on the edge dislocations $XY$ and $AB$ in Fig. 7.2 are parallel to the Burgers vectors of the dislocation and therefore have a *screw orientation*. The jogs lie in the slip plane of the main dislocation so that they will not impede the motion of the edge dislocations. Thus, an important conclusion is that *jogs in pure edge dislocations do not affect the subsequent motion of the dislocation*.

Consider the jogs in the screw dislocations in Figs. 7.3 and 7.4. All the jogs have an *edge character*. Since an edge dislocation can glide freely only in the plane containing its line and Burgers vector, the only way the jog can move by slip, i.e. *conservatively*, is along the axis of the screw dislocation as illustrated in Fig. 7.5. Therefore, the screw dislocation can move forward and take the jog with it only by a *non-conservative process*. This process requires thermal activation and consequently the movement of the screw dislocation will be tempera-

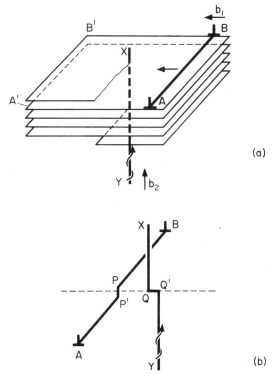

FIG. 7.3. Intersection of an edge dislocation with a right-handed screw dislocation. (a) A dislocation *AB* moving in its slip plane is about to cut a screw dislocation *XY*. The crystal consists of a single spiral surface. *AB* glides over this surface and after crossing the screw dislocation the ends *A'* and *B'* will not lie on the same plane. Thus the dislocation must contain a jog *PP'* as show in (b). (After READ (1953), *Dislocations in Crystals*, McGraw-Hill.)

ture dependent. At a sufficiently high stress, movement of the jog will leave behind a trail of vacancies or interstitial atoms depending on the sign of the dislocation and the direction the dislocation is moving. A jog which moves in such a direction that it produces vacancies is called a *vacancy jog*, and if it moves in the opposite direction it is called an *interstitial jog*.

So far only single jogs on screw dislocations have been considered. In practice the screw dislocation will "collect" a lot of jogs during its

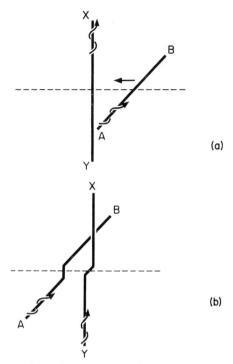

FIG. 7.4. Intersection of screw dislocations. (a) Before intersection.
(b) After intersection.

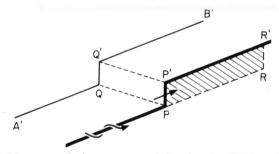

FIG. 7.5. Movement of a jog on a screw dislocation. Jog *PP'* has a Burgers
vector normal to *PP'* and is, therefore, a short length of edge dislocation.
The plane defined by *PP'* and its Burgers vector is *PP'RR'* and is the plane
in which *PP'* can glide. Movement of the screw dislocation to *A'QQ'B'* would
require climb of the jog along *PQ*.

movement through the forest dislocations. Both vacancy and interstitial jogs will be formed and these will tend to glide (Fig. 7.5) in
opposite directions along the dislocation and annihilate each other.
This will result in a net concentration of jogs all of the same sign and,
because of their mutual repulsion, they will be approximately evenly
spaced along the dislocation line. Consider a pure screw dislocation
*AB* in Fig. 7.6 with a uniformly spaced array of vacancy jogs along
its length. The jogs will act as pinning points on the dislocation so
that, under an applied shear stress $\tau$ acting in the slip direction, the
dislocation will *bow out* between the jogs (Fig. 7.6(b)). The radius of
curvature $\varrho$ of the dislocation due to the shear stress is given by
equation (4.19). There will be a critical stage, radius of curvature $\varrho_c$,
at which the stress required to produce further bowing out of the
dislocation is greater than that required to produce vacancies at the
jog so that the dislocation will move forward leaving a trail of vacancies behind each jog (Fig. 7.6(c)).

According to Seeger (1954), the energy required to form a vacancy
or an interstitial atom at the jog may be written

$$U_1 = \alpha_1 Gb^3 \qquad (7.1)$$

where $\alpha_1$ is approximately equal to 1 for an interstitial atom and is
between 0·1 nd 0·2 for a vacancy in face-centred cubic metals, i.e.
taking $G = 30$ GN m$^{-2}$ and $b = 0·3$ nm, $U_1$ is 0·8 aJ and 0·1 aJ for
an interstitial atom and vacancy respectively. When all the jogs move
forward by one atom spacing, due to the formation of vacancies or
interstitial atoms, the whole dislocation will move forward one spacing. Thus, if $x$ is the spacing between jogs, the work done on the dislocation will be

$$W = \tau b^2 x \qquad (7.2)$$

for each length of dislocation associated with a jog. Equating (7.1)
and (7.2) the shear stress required to generate a defect and move the
dislocation in the absence of thermal activation will be

$$\tau = \alpha_1 \frac{Gb}{x} . \qquad (7.3)$$

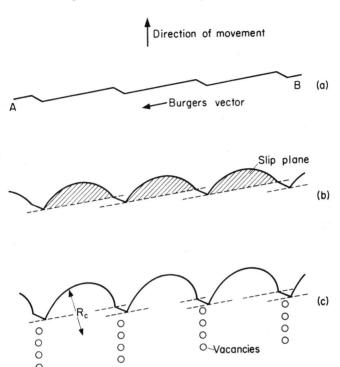

FIG. 7.6. Movement of a jogged screw dislocation. (a) Straight dislocation under zero stress. (b) Dislocation bowed out in the slip plane between the jogs due to applied shear stress. (c) Movement of dislocation leaving trails of vacancies behind the jogs.

At elevated temperatures thermal activation assists in the formation of a vacancy, and the activation energy $U_{(\tau)}$ for movement of the jog, or the formation of defects at the jog, will be given by

$$U_{(\tau)} = \alpha_1 Gb^3 - \tau b^2 x. \qquad (7.4)$$

Since $\alpha_1$ is much larger for interstitial atoms than for vacancies, vacancy formation will occur more readily than interstitial atom formation. The condition in equation (7.4) is readily satisfied for elementary vacancy jogs on dislocations in body-centred cubic and face-centred cubic metals but it is doubtful whether or not interstitial atoms can be formed at interstitial jogs. There is a considerable volume of experimental evidence which shows that vacancies are produced by the movement of dislocations during plastic deformation. The usual method is to compare the changes in physical properties, such as electrical resistivity, which are produced by quenching from elevated temperatures with those produced by plastic deformation.

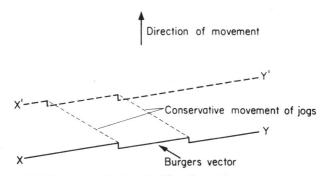

Fig. 7.7. Movement of a jogged dislocation with a screw component without the formation of point defects. *XY* initial position, *X'Y'* final position.

It can be assumed with confidence that the change in resistivity, produced by quenching and subsequent annealing, results directly from the introduction and removal of vacancies. Similar changes occur after plastic deformation.

It is possible for a dislocation with jogs to glide without producing defects. Consider the dislocation *XY* (Fig. 7.7), with a Burgers vector not parallel to the main dislocation line, moving in the direction indicated. As the dislocation moves forward the jogs can glide conservatively along the dislocation tracing the path indicated by the dotted lines. Whether or not this occurs in preference to the non-conservative motion of the jogs will depend on the relative ease with which the two processes occur.

## 7.4 Composite Jogs

Any jog more than one atomic plane spacing high is referred to as a *composite jog*. The movement of dislocations with composite jogs can be divided into three groups depending on the height of the jog. These are illustrated in Fig. 7.8 after Gilman and Johnston (1962). For very small jogs (Fig. 7.8(a)) with heights of 1 or 2 atom spacings, the screw dislocation will drag the jog along creating point defects as described in section 7.3. For very large jogs, where the distance between the two dislocation segments is large enough to

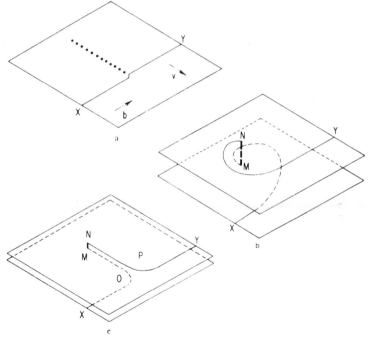

FIG. 7.8. Behaviour of jogs with different heights on a screw dislocation. (a) Small jog is dragged along, creating point defects as it moves. (b) Very large jog—the dislocations *NY* and *XM* move independently. (c) Intermediate jog—the dislocations *NP* and *MO* interact and cannot pass by one another except at a high stress. (From GILMAN and JOHNSTON, *Solid State Physics*, **13**, 147, 1962.)

prevent their mutual interaction, the dislocations will behave separately as single ended sources (see Chapter 8 on dislocation multiplication). The separation required for this type of behaviour can be estimated by calculating the maximum interaction stress between two parallel edge dislocations of opposite sign and comparing this with the effective applied stress. Before the dislocations can expand into the position illustrated in Fig. 7.8(b) they must pass an intermediate position similar to that illustrated in Fig. 7.8(c). In this orientation the lengths *NP* and *MO* are pure edge dislocations of opposite sign. The maximum force between two dislocations of opposite sign can be obtained directly from Fig. 4.8, i.e.

$$F_{x\,max} = \frac{0 \cdot 25Gb^2}{2\pi(1-\nu)\,y} \tag{7.5}$$

where $y$ is the spacing between the two planes, or the height of the jog *NM*. Since $F_x = \tau b$ (equation (4.16)) the dislocation interaction stress will be

$$\tau = \frac{0 \cdot 25Gb}{2\pi(1-\nu)\,y}. \tag{7.6}$$

Taking some typical values for a silicon iron (Low and Turkalo, 1962), $G = 58$ GN m$^{-2}$, $b = 0 \cdot 25$ nm, $\nu = 0 \cdot 3$, and $\tau = 45$ MN m$^{-2}$ it is found that $y \approx 20$n m. Thus, providing the jog height is greater than 20 nm, the two segments can pass each other under the applied stress and operate independently. Jogs of intermediate size will result in the arrangement shown in Fig. 7.8(c), consisting of a trail of two edge dislocations with the same Burgers vector but of opposite sign. This arrangement is called a *dislocation dipole*.

Examples of these three types of jog are shown in Fig. 7.9. This is an electron transmission micrograph of a thin foil prepared from a slice of crystal carefully cut from a large silicon iron single crystal after it had been deformed about 1 per cent. Slip occurred on only one slip system, namely, (011) [$\bar{1}\bar{1}1$], and the slice was cut parallel to the (011) slip plane. The [$\bar{1}\bar{1}1$] and [$2\bar{1}1$] directions in the (011) plane of the foil are marked on the photograph. Since the Burgers

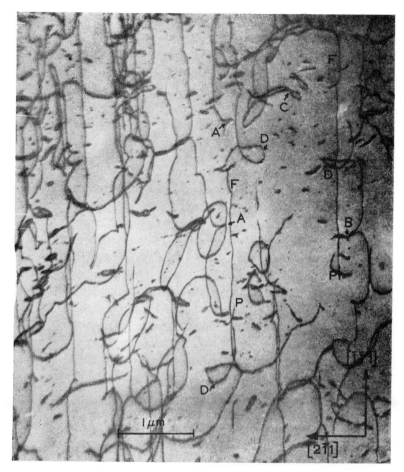

FIG. 7.9. Transmission micrograph of thin foil of iron 3 per cent silicon alloy parallel to (011) slip plane. *A*, dipole trails. *B* and *C* pinching off of dipole trails. *D* single ended sources at large jogs. *FP* jogged screw dislocation. (From Low and TURKALO, *Acta Met.* **10**, 215, 1962.)

vector of the slip dislocations in body-centred cubic metals is of the type $\frac{1}{2}\langle 111 \rangle$ all the segments of dislocations parallel to [$\bar{1}\bar{1}1$] will be pure screw dislocations and segments normal to [$\bar{1}\bar{1}1$], i.e. parallel to [$2\bar{1}1$] will be edge dislocations. The screw dislocations are relatively

long and have numerous jogs along their length, e.g. the dislocations
*FP*. Examples of dislocation dipoles occur at points *A* and they are
aligned approximately in the [2Ī1] edge orientation as expected.
Single ended sources have been produced at site *D*.

A ready source of composite jogs is double cross slip which is
illustrated in Fig. 3.8. The segments of the dislocation which do not
lie in the principal slip plane have a predominantly edge character.
More generally, any movement of the dislocation out of the slip
plane will result in the formation of jogs. This is particularly important
in body-centred cubic metals where the slip plane is often not well
defined, and the screw dislocations tend to move on the plane of maximum resolved shear stress rather than on a specific crystallographic
plane. It is more difficult to produce jogs in crystals with extended
dislocations because slip on a cross slip plane is restricted.

In many cases cross slip is unlikely unless local stress concentrations
are present and this led Tetelman (1962) to propose an alternative
mechanism for the formation of dipoles. The sequence of events is
illustrated in Fig. 7.10. Two non-parallel dislocations *MM'* and
*NN'* are gliding in parallel slip planes separated by a distance *y* (Fig.
7.10(a)). If the Burgers vectors of the dislocations are equal but of
opposite sign, the dislocations can lower their energy by reorientating
part of their lengths in the glide plane, as in Fig. 7.10(b). The segments
*PP'* and *RR'* are predominantly edge dislocations and will lie approximately above each other. Under an applied shear stress *PP'* and *RR'*
will attempt to separate in their glide planes. This situation is similar
to the crossing over of edge dislocation segments on each side of a
large jog (Fig. 7.8) and the dislocations will interact strongly with
each other if the spacing between the planes is small (equation 7.5).
Thus, depending on the applied stress and spacing of the slip planes,
the dislocations will not cross and the arrangement in Fig. 7.10(b)
will be stable. However, if either the dislocation *P'M'* or *R'N* is close
to a pure screw orientation, part of it (say *P'M'*) can cross slip down
and join the dislocation *R'N* at *R'*. Since *P'M'* and *R'N* have opposite
Burgers vectors the cross slip segment will be annihilated leaving a
dislocation dipole *MPP'R'RN'*. The dislocation *NTT'M'* in Fig.

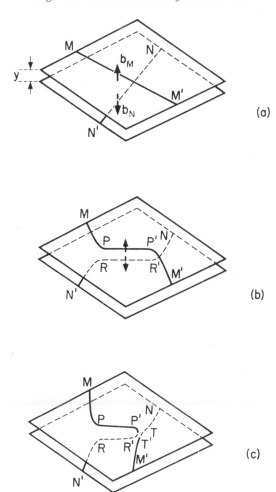

FIG. 7.10. Mechanism for dislocation dipole formation. (After Tetelman, *Acta Met.* **10,** 813, 1962.)

7.10(c) will have a jog $TT'$ and will move according to the description given above for composite jogs. This mechanism accounts for the formation of dipoles in the very early stages of plastic deformation where slip is confined to one set of slip planes.

## 7.5 Jogs and Prismatic Loops

Trails of defects and prismatic loops are often produced during plastic deformation. In Fig. 7.9 numerous small loops, many of them elongated, can be seen. Prior to deformation, the specimen in this photograph had a very low dislocation density and there were no loops present. This so-called *debris* is left behind by moving dislocations and is a direct result of edge jogs on screw dislocations.

Two mechanisms of forming loops are possible. Firstly, by the diffusion and coalescence of vacancies formed at a moving jog, thus consider an elementary jog leaving a single trail of defects; if the temperature is sufficiently high to allow diffusion of the defects they will collect together and form a vacancy or interstitial platelet which will then form a dislocation loop (sections 5.5. and 6.4). At low temperatures interstitials diffuse more readily than vacancies and providing interstitials can be formed at an elementary jog, it will be possible to form interstitial dislocation loops. Vacancy loops, however, form only at higher temperatures because of the restricted rate of diffusion. The second mechanism represents a further stage in the movement of a dislocation dipole formed either from an intermediate sized jog (Fig. 7.8(c)) or by the interaction of dislocations on parallel slip planes (Fig. 7.10). The dipole can break up and lower its overall elastic energy by forming a row of prismatic loops. Two stages in this process are illustrated in Fig. 7.11. An elongated loop is formed which then breaks up into isolated loops. This may occur partly

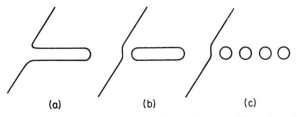

(a)             (b)            (c)

FIG. 7.11. Formation of dislocation loops from a dislocation dipole. (a) Dislocation dipole. (b) Elongated loop and jogged dislocation. (c) Row of small loops.

by a cross slip mechanism similar to the pinching off of dislocations $P'M'$ and $R'N$ in Fig. 7.10(b). The pinching off of dipoles can be seen at points $C$ in Fig. 7.9. The formation of a row of loops from a long elongated dipole is shown in Fig. 7.12. The dislocations are SA/TB type dislocations (see section 6.2) formed during plastic deformation of cadmium at about $-100°C$. A long dipole $AB$ is in the process of splitting up, and at $D$ a long loop is splitting into two circular loops. A row of loops can be seen at the top of the photograph. Although these changes occurred at low temperatures they are thought to involve pipe diffusion along the dislocations which can result in the redistribution of material close to the loop (section 3.8). The activation energy for pipe diffusion is lower than that of volume self-diffusion. The dislocation loops formed by the breaking up of dipoles can be either vacancy or interstitial loops depending on the sign of the initial jog or dipole.

### 7.6 Intersections of Extended Dislocations

The simple geometrical models of intersections illustrated in Figs. 7.2–7.5 have to be modified somewhat when the intersecting dislocations are extended, as is expected to be the case in face-centred cubic metals with low stacking fault energies. It is difficult to generalise the problem because of the number of variants of intersections that are possible. One example will be considered to illustrate some of the principles involved. In Fig. 7.13 two extended dislocations intersect at right angles. The dislocations can only cut through each other by constricting to form unit unextended dislocations in the region close to the intersection (Fig. 7.13(b)). The dislocations can then separate and elementary jogs are produced on the extended dislocations (Fig. 7.13(c)). It is clear that to form jogs on extended dislocations work will have to be done to constrict the dislocations and so the energy of the jog will depend on the stacking fault energy or, alternatively, on the spacing of the partial dislocations. Estimates of the jog energy have been made by Stroh (1954), Seeger (1954) and Friedel (1964).

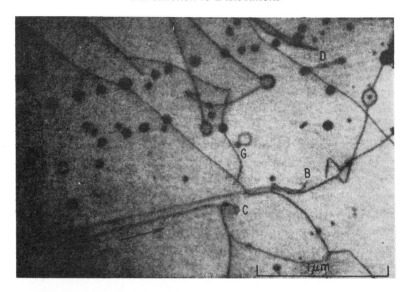

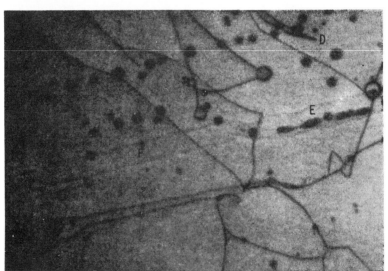

FIG. 7.12. Transmission electron micrographs, taken with a 30-sec interval, of a cadmium (0001) platelet at $-95°C$ showing dislocation dipoles and the splitting up of long sessile loops. (From PRICE, *J. Appl. Phys.* **32**, 1750, 1961.)

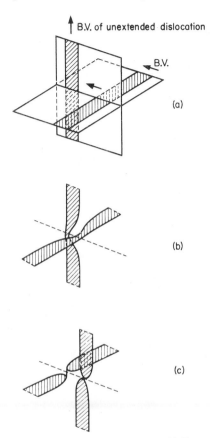

Fig. 7.13. Intersection of extended dislocations. (a) Extended dislocations moving towards each other, but separated by a large distance. (b) Constriction of dislocations due to the interaction of the elastic strain fields of the leading partial dislocations. (c) Formation of jogs on extended dislocations.

## 7.7 Extended Jogs

The description of the movement of dislocations containing jogs in section 7.3 showed that jogs in screw dislocations can move conservatively only by glide along the axis of the screw dislocation, whereas jogs in edge dislocations can move conservatively only by glide in the direction of dislocation movement. The situation is more complicated when the jog segment of the dislocation can lower its energy by dissociating into partial dislocations, because the jog will have to constrict before it can glide. Depending on the nature of the jog and the way it dissociates, two situations can be envisaged. (a) The applied stress is sufficient to constrict the jog and allow it to glide conservatively. (b) The applied stress is insufficient to constrict the jog, which will be sessile, but greater than that required to cause individual segments of the dislocation to bow out and form dislocation dipoles. These problems have been considered in detail by Hirsch (1962) for all the possible jog configurations in face-centred cubic metals.

## 7.8 Attractive and Repulsive Junctions

In section 4.6 it was shown that parallel edge dislocations of opposite sign lying on the same slip plane attracted each other by a force given by equation (4.23) whereas edge dislocations of the same sign repelled each other with an equal but opposite force. In the same way a dislocation crossing a *forest* dislocation will interact with the elastic stress field of the latter and will be attracted or repelled depending on the Burgers vector of the dislocations and the angle $\phi$ between the intersecting dislocation lines.

Consider a straight dislocation $LL'$ crossing a second dislocation $MM'$, as in Fig. 7.14. The stress field of $LL'$ will interact with $MM'$ over a short length which will increase as $\phi$ decreases. If the distance separating the dislocations is $r$, the stress field of $MM'$ can be considered to act on a length $\pi r \cos \phi$ of $LL'$. If the stress field of $MM'$ tends to repel $LL'$, work will be done in moving $LL'$ until it intersects $MM'$ in addition to the work necessary to form a jog; this is called a *repulsive junction*. If the stress field of $MM'$ attracts $LL'$ energy will be required to separate the dislocations after they have intersected; this is called an *attractive junction*.

For dislocations which intersect rigidly, as illustrated in Figs. 7.2–7.5, repulsive and attractive junctions may be considered to be equal and opposite because one can be obtained from the other by changing the sign of a Burgers vector. However, because dislocations are flexible, they will bend as they approach each other to lower the energy at the intersection as much as possible. The reduction in energy

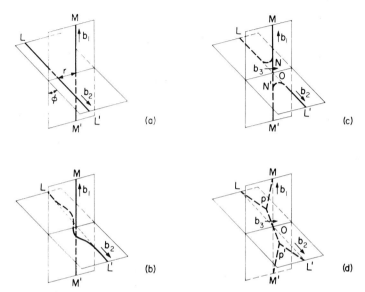

FIG. 7.14. Illustration of an attractive junction. (a) Dislocation $LL'$ moves toward $MM'$. If the angle $2\theta$ between $\mathbf{b}_1$ and $\mathbf{b}_2$ is $> \frac{1}{2}\pi$ the dislocations attract each other, and if $2\theta < \frac{1}{2}\pi$ the dislocations repel each other. (b) (c) and (d) $LL'$ and $MM'$ react to form a new dislocation $PP'$.

is equivalent to an attraction, which for an attractive junction will strengthen the attraction, but for a repulsive junction will reduce the repulsion. The attractive junctions are therefore stronger.

The stress required to complete the intersection of a repulsive junction, ignoring the stress to form a jog, can be calculated from the work done in moving the dislocations together. The simplest example is the intersection of pure screws, as illustrated in Fig. 7.14, and can be calculated following Carrington, Hale and McLean, 1960 (*Proc. Roy. Soc.* A, **259**, 203, 1960). The Burgers vectors of dislocations $LL'$ and $MM'$ are $\mathbf{b}_1$ and $\mathbf{b}_2$ and they lie at an angle $2\theta$ to each other. If $b_1 = b_2 = b$, the force acting on length $\pi r \cos \phi$ will be

$$F_r = \frac{Gb^2}{2\pi r} \cos 2\theta \cdot \pi r \cos \phi$$

$$= \frac{Gb^2}{2} \cos 2\theta \cos \phi. \qquad (7.7)$$

If the distance between intersecting forest dislocations of the type $MM'$ is $x$, an applied stress $\tau_r$ acting on a length $x$ does work $\tau_r b^2 x$ as the dislocation moves forward a distance $b$ against the force $F_r$. Equating the work done,

$$F_r b = \tau_r b^2 x. \qquad (7.8)$$

Substitution in (7.7) gives

$$\tau_r = \frac{Gb}{x} \frac{\cos 2\theta \cos \phi}{2}. \qquad (7.9)$$

Taking a specific example of screw dislocations in body-centred cubic metals $2\theta = \phi = 109 \cdot 5°$ gives

$$\tau_r = \frac{0 \cdot 056 \, Gb}{x}. \qquad (7.10)$$

It is expected that all repulsive junctions will give values of this order of magnitude. This is much smaller than the stress to make jogs, i.e. from section 7.3, $\tau \simeq \alpha_1 \, Gb/x$, where $\alpha_1 = 0 \cdot 2$ for vacancy jogs, and, therefore, *repulsive junctions* make only a small contribution to the stress required to move dislocations.

A particularly large reduction in energy at an attractive junction can result when a dislocation reaction occurs which reduces the total length of dislocation line. The sequence of events is illustrated in Fig. 7.14 for the intersection of two screw dislocations. Dislocation $LL'$ moves towards $MM'$. Assume for simplicity that $MM'$ is inflexible but that $LL'$ is free to glide but not to climb. When $LL'$ is close to $MM'$ it is attracted and tends to align itself parallel to $MM'$ over part of its length (Fig. 7.14(b)). The two dislocations then react to produce a third dislocation $NN'$ with Burgers vector $\mathbf{b}_3$

$$\mathbf{b}_1 + \mathbf{b}_2 \rightarrow \mathbf{b}_3 \tag{7.11}$$

as shown in Fig. 7.14(c). For this reaction to be energetically favourable

$$b_1^2 + b_2^2 > b_3^2. \tag{7.12}$$

If the strengths of the dislocation are equal this condition is satisfied if the angle between the Burgers vectors $2\theta > \frac{1}{2}\pi$. A further small reduction in energy occurs when the dislocations take up equilibrium positions (Fig. 7.14(d)), determined by the condition that the dislocation line length is a minimum. If the dislocations in Fig. 7.14(d) are assumed to be pinned, for example, by other forest dislocations, at $L$, $M$, $M'$ and $L'$ the reduction in energy at the intersection will be approximately given by

$$E = 2[(LO + OM)\, W_1 - (LP + PM)\, W_1 - OP\, W_3], \tag{7.13}$$

where $W_1$ is the energy per unit length of $LO$, $OM$, $LP$ and $PM$ and $W_3$ is the energy per unit length of $PP'$. Carrington, Hale and McLean calculated the stress required to push a dislocation through a forest of attractive junctions by calculating the work done in changing the configuration of the dislocations from the minimum energy position $LPP'L'$ and $MPP'M'$ to position $LOL'$ and $MOM'$. For attractive junctions in body-centred cubic metals it was found that,

$$\tau_j = \frac{0 \cdot 22\, Gb}{x} \tag{7.14}$$

where $x$ is the spacing of forest dislocations, and for face-centred cubic metals,

$$\tau_j = \frac{0 \cdot 33\, Gb}{x}. \tag{7.15}$$

Since jogs are formed at attractive junctions an additional stress is required to separate the dislocations. By symmetry, only half the jog energy must be provided at separation and therefore the additional stress will be approximately $0.1\ Gb/x$.

## 7.9 Measurement of Stacking Fault Energy in Face-centred Cubic Metals

A particularly interesting dislocation reaction, which provides a method for the direct experimental measurement of stacking fault energy, is illustrated in Fig. 7.15. When a dislocation on a plane α

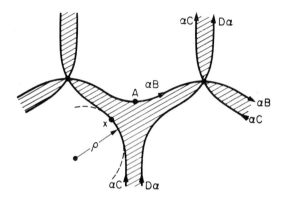

Fig. 7.15. Extended node in a face-centred cubic lattice. The shaded area represents a stacking fault. (From Whelan, *Proc. Roy. Soc.* A, **249**, 114, 1959.)

with a Burgers vector **DC** (Thompson notation) intersects a dislocation on plane δ with a Burgers vector **CB**, the resulting arrangement of dislocation can be represented by Fig. 7.15. Initially **DC** is dissociated into **Dα + αC** and **CB** into **Cδ + δB**. The dislocations constrict at the intersection and then **CB** dissociates into plane α to form **Cα + αB**. A network of contracted and extended nodes formed during deformation of a copper–8 per cent aluminium alloy at room temperature is shown in Fig. 7.16.

The partial dislocation at $X$ (in Fig. 7.15) is in equilibrium under (i) a force $F$ per unit length, tending to straighten the line, due to the line energy $T$ and curvature of the dislocation $\varrho$, given by

$$F = \frac{T}{\varrho} \qquad (7.16)$$

where $T$ is given in equation (4.17) and (ii) a force $\gamma$ per unit length, tending to contract the node, due to the attraction produced by the stacking fault, where $\gamma$ is the stacking fault energy. Equating these forces

$$\gamma = \frac{T}{\varrho} \simeq \frac{\alpha G b^2}{\varrho} . \qquad (7.17)$$

No account has been taken in this relation of the interaction energy of nearby partial dislocations, and of the variation of line tension along the curved dislocation. However, bearing these limitations in mind, the stacking fault energy can be determined directly from

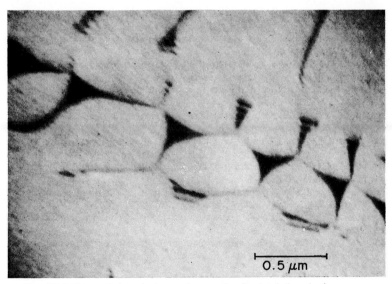

FIG. 7.16. Transmission electron micrograph of extended nodes in a copper–8 per cent aluminium alloy deformed 5 per cent at room temperature. (From SWANN (1963), *Electron Microscopy and Strength of Crystals*, p. 131, Interscience.)

equation (7.17) providing $\varrho$ can be measured. In practice, the method is limited to solids with low stacking fault energies because of the difficulty of measuring $\varrho$. Thus, the stacking fault energy of pure face-centred cubic metals are difficult to measure, but the method is readily applied to face-centred cubic metal alloys and many of the layer structures.

*Further Reading*

CARRINGTON, W., HALE, K. F. and McLEAN, D. (1960) "Arrangement of dislocations in iron", *Proc. Roy. Soc.* A, **259**, 203.

COTTRELL, A. H. (1958) "Point defects and mechanical properties", *Vacancies and Other Point Defects in Metal and Alloys*, Inst. Metals, London.

FRIEDEL. J. (1964) *Dislocations*, Pergamon Press, Oxford.

GILMAN, J. J. and JOHNSTON, W. G. (1962) "Dislocations in lithium fluoride", *Solid State Physics*, **13**, 147.

HIRSCH, P. B. (1962) "Extended jogs in face-centred cubic metals", *Phil. Mag.* **7**, 67.

HIRTH, J. P. and LOTHE, J. (1966) "Glide of jogged dislocations", *Can. J. Phys.* **45**, 809.

HOWIE, A. and SWANN, P. R. (1961) "Direct measurements of stacking fault energies", *Phil. Mag.* **6**, 1215.

LOW, J. R. and TURKALO, A. M. (1962) "Slip band structure and dislocation multiplication in silicon iron crystals", *Acta Metall.* **10**, 215.

PRICE, P. B. (1961) "Non-basal glide in cadmium crystals", *J. Appl. Phys.* **32**, 1750.

SEEGER, A. (1955) "Jogs in dislocation lines," *Defects in Crystalline Solids*, p. 391, Physical Society, London.

SEITZ, F. (1952) "Generation of vacancies by moving dislocations", *Adv. Physics*, **1**, 43.

STROH, A. N. (1954) "Constriction of jogs in extended dislocations", *Proc. Phys. Soc.* (London), B **67**, 427.

SWANN, P. R. (1963) "Dislocation arrangements in face-centred cubic metals", *Electron Microscopy and Strength of Crystals*, p. 131, Wiley.

TETELMAN, A. S. (1962) "Dislocation dipole formation in deformed crystals", *Acta Metall.* **10**, 813.

WHELAN, M. J. (1959) "Dislocation interactions in face-centred cubic metals", *Proc. Roy. Soc.* A, **249**, 114.

CHAPTER 8

# Origin and Multiplication of Dislocations

## 8.1 Introduction

Apart from crystal *whiskers* and isolated examples in larger crystals of materials like silicon, dislocations occur in all crystals. The dislocation density in well-annealed crystals (i.e. crystals which have been heated for a long time close to their melting point to reduce the dislocation density to a low value) is usually about $10^6$ cm$^{-2}$ and the dislocations are arranged in networks as previously mentioned in Chapter 1 (Fig. 1.19). A similar density of dislocations is present in crystals immediately after they have been grown from the melt or produced by strain anneal techniques and the origin of these dislocations is described in the next section.

When annealed crystals are deformed there is a rapid multiplication of dislocations and a progressive increase in dislocation density with increasing strain. After large amounts of plastic deformation the dislocation density is typically in the range $10^{10}$ to $10^{11}$ cm$^{-2}$. In the early stages of deformation dislocation movement tends to be confined to a single set of parallel slip planes. Later, slip occurs on other slip systems and dislocations moving on different systems interact. The rapid multiplication leads to work hardening (Chapter 10). In this chapter the main mechanisms of dislocation multiplication will be described.

## 8.2 Dislocations in Freshly Grown Crystals

It is very difficult to grow crystals with low dislocation densities because dislocations are readily introduced during the growing process. There are two main sources of dislocations in freshly grown crystals. Firstly, dislocations or other defects present in the "seed" crystals or other surfaces used to initiate the growth of the crystal. Any dislocations in a seed crystal which intersect the surface of the seed on which new growth occurs will extend into the growing crystal. Secondly, "accidental" nucleation during the growth process. The main mechanisms which have been suggested are: (a) heterogeneous nucleation of dislocations due to internal stresses generated by impurity particles, thermal contraction, etc.; (b) impingement of different parts of the growing interface; (c) formation and subsequent movement of dislocation loops formed by the collapse of vacancy platelets.

The basic principle involved in the nucleation of dislocations by local internal stresses during growth and subsequent cooling is embodied in the specific example given in section 8.4. High local internal stresses are produced when neighbouring parts of the crystal are constrained to change their specific volume. This can occur by neighbouring regions expanding or contracting by different amounts due to (a) thermal gradients, (b) change in composition, or (c) change in lattice structure. An additional effect is the adherence of the growing crystal to the sides of the container. When the stress reaches a critical value, about $G/30$, dislocations are nucleated. If this occurs at high temperatures the dislocations created will rearrange themselves by climb. It should also be noted that under normal laboratory conditions there is every possibility of isolated vibrations which will affect the growth process and produce additional random stress effects.

The formation of dislocations by impingement is most clearly demonstrated during the coalescence of two adjacent dendrites in the growing interface. Thus, the dendrites may be misaligned or have growth steps on their surfaces so that perfect matching is impossible and dislocations are formed at the interfaces.

The formation of dislocation loops by collapse of vacancy platelets follows directly from previous descriptions of the formation of dislocation loops. In section 1.5 it was shown that, when crystals are rapidly cooled from temperatures close to the melting point, the high-temperature equilibrium concentration of vacancies is retained in a supersaturated state and the vacancies can precipitate to form dislocation loops. A critical supersaturation $c_1$ is required for the process. This is illustrated by the fact that, in quenched specimens containing a sufficient supersaturation of vacancies to form loops in the centre of grains, no loops are found close to grain boundaries because the degree of supersaturation is reduced by the migration of vacancies to the boundary. The solidification of a melt involves the movement of a liquid–solid interface. There is normally an appreciable temperature gradient in the solid. Immediately below the interface the solid will be very close to the melting point and the equilibrium concentration of vacancies will be high. If this region cools sufficiently rapidly a high density of vacancies will be retained and, providing the supersaturation is greater than $c_1$, loops will be formed. Speculation about this mechanism revolves around whether or not the supersaturation is sufficient. It is most unlikely to be so when the rate of cooling is slow. However, any loops that are produced in the solid phase below the moving interface will expand by climb due to diffusion of vacancies to the loop. Loops formed at a large angle to the interface may eventually intersect the interface and the two points of emergence formed in this way will act as a site for the propagation of dislocations into the new crystal.

### 8.3 Homogeneous Nucleation of Dislocations

When a dislocation is created in a region of the crystal that is free from any defects the nucleation is referred to as *homogeneous*. This occurs only under extreme conditions because a very large stress is required. A method of estimating the stress has been described by Cottrell (1953). Imagine that two parallel screw dislocations, of opposite sense, are nucleated in a crystal by an applied stress and begin to move apart. The force on each of them is $\tau b$, and if they move a distance $S$ apart they do work equal to $\tau bS$ per unit length. From equation (4.9) the energy of each dislocation is $E_{(S)} = (Gb^2/4\pi)\ln(R/r_0)$, and in this example $R = S$ because the strain due to each dislocation is cancelled by the other one at large distances compared with $S$. Thus, the total change in energy of the crystal is

$$E_T = \frac{Gb^2}{4\pi}\ln\frac{S}{r_0} - \tau bS. \qquad (8.1)$$

This energy is zero for $S = 0$, rises to a maximum at a certain value of $S = S^*$, and then drops to zero and becomes negative. At the energy maximum

$$\frac{dE_T}{dS} = 0 = \frac{Gb^2}{4\pi}\frac{1}{S^*} - \tau b,$$

therefore

$$S^* = \frac{Gb}{4\pi\tau}. \qquad (8.2)$$

Taking $r_0 \approx b$, the energy maximum $E_T^*$ is

$$E_T^* = \frac{Gb^2}{4\pi}\left(\ln\frac{G}{4\pi\tau} - 1\right). \qquad (8.3)$$

For spontaneous nucleation $E_T^*$ must be reduced to zero by the applied stress, i.e.

$$\ln\frac{G}{4\pi\tau} - 1 = 0. \qquad (8.4)$$

Thus the stress, $\tau_N$, required is

$$\tau_N = \frac{G}{4\pi e} \simeq \frac{G}{30}. \qquad (8.5)$$

This stress is much higher than the uniform stress at which materials normally deform plastically which implies that other processes, such as the movement of existing dislocations, are preferred. However, it is possible that strain concentrations will raise the stress to this level in local volumes of the crystal.

### 8.4 Nucleation of Dislocations at Stress Concentrators

A well-known example of the nucleation of dislocations at a stress concentration is illustrated in Fig. 8.1. Spherical glass inclusions were introduced into a crystal of silver chloride which was subsequently

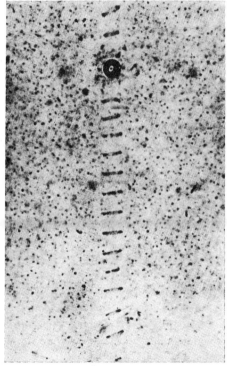

FIG. 8.1. System of prismatic dislocation loops produced in a recrystallised, dislocation-free, crystal of silver chloride to relax the strain field around the small glass sphere caused by differential contraction which occurs during cooling. (From MITCHELL (1958), *Growth and Perfection of Crystals*, p. 386, Wiley.)

given a treatment to reduce the dislocation density to a low value. The crystal was held at 370°C to homogenise the temperature, and remove any internal strains associated with the inclusion, and then cooled to 20°C. The dislocations were revealed by a decoration technique (section 2.3). The photograph shows a row of prismatic dislocation loops, viewed edge on, which have been *punched out* from around the glass inclusion during cooling. The axis of the loops is parallel to a $\langle 110 \rangle$ direction which is the principal slip direction in this structure. The nucleation of the dislocation results from the stress produced around the sphere by the differential contraction of the crystal and the glass inclusion during cooling. Suppose that at 370°C the inclusion has unit radius; it will be resting in a hole in the silver chloride also of unit radius. If the coefficient of expansion of glass and silver chloride are $\alpha_1$ and $\alpha_2$ respectively, and $\alpha_1 < \alpha_2$, then on cooling to 20°C the natural radius of the inclusion will be $1 - 350\alpha_1$ and the natural radius of the hole will be $1 - 350\alpha_2$. If the inclusion is unyielding this will result in a spherically symmetrical strain field in the surrounding matrix which can be estimated by analogy with the strain field around a spherical hole with an internal pressure. Thus, consider a particle of radius $r(1 + \varepsilon)$ in a hole of natural radius $r$ in an infinite isotropic elastic medium; $\varepsilon$ is termed the misfit parameter. The radial displacement of a particle at a distance $R$, for $R > r$ is

$$\varepsilon_R = \varepsilon \left( \frac{r}{R} \right)^3. \tag{8.6}$$

The maximum shear stress produced in the matrix, resolved parallel to a given radial direction (the specific direction is immaterial because of the spherical symmetry), lies at the surface of the spherical inclusion on a cylindrical surface of diameter $r_1\sqrt{2}$, where $r_1$ is the diameter of the inclusion. This is illustrated in section in Fig. 8.2. The magnitude of the stress is

$$\tau_{max} = 3\varepsilon G \tag{8.7}$$

Taking $\alpha_1 = 34 \times 10^{-7}$ for the glass particle and $\alpha_2 = 345 \times 10^{-7}$ for the silver chloride crystal gives $\varepsilon \simeq 0.01$ after the crystal and inclusion

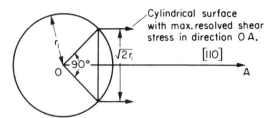

FIG. 8.2. Section of spherical particle.

have cooled to 20°C and

$$\tau_{max} = \frac{G}{33}. \tag{8.8}$$

This is close to the stress required to nucleate dislocations. The dislocations formed in this way at the interface will move away under the influence of the strain field of the inclusion.

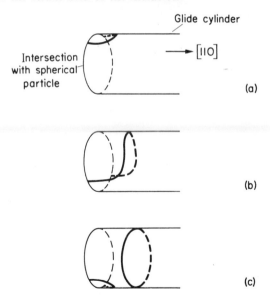

FIG. 8.3. Mechanism of formation of prismatic loops around and inclusion. (a) Small loop at the surface of inclusion. (b) Loop expands around glide cylinder. (c) Prismatic loop.

The mechanism for formation of the loops is as follows. The preferred slip vectors in silver chloride are of the type $\frac{1}{2}\langle 110\rangle$. Under the action of $\tau_{max}$ in the [110] direction a small loop forms on the surface of the glide cylinder indicated in Fig. 8.3. The forward edge component glides away from the interface under the influence of a stress field which decreases in intensity with increasing distance from the interface. The screw components of the loop, which are parallel to the axis of the glide cylinder, experience a tangential force which causes them to glide in opposite directions around the surface of the cylinder. The dislocation must retain its screw orientation at the interface but elsewhere it will become inclined to the axis as it glides round the cylinder and the dislocation develops a mixed edge–screw character.

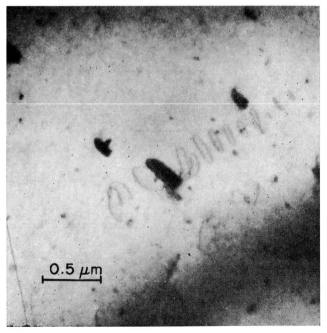

FIG. 8.4. Transmission electron micrograph of prismatic loops punched out at a carbide precipitate in iron. The precipitate formed during cooling. (From MOGFORD and HULL (1959), unpublished.)

Its movement is restricted to the glide cylinder because any radial displacement requires climb. When the two ends of the loop, which rotate around the axis under the action of the tangential stress, intersect, a dislocation loop will be produced. This is a positive prismatic dislocation loop and as it moves away along the [110] axis it is effectively moving material away from the inclusion and so relaxing the strain field. The process can be repeated to produce a series of loops. More complex patterns are obtained when the glide cylinders of the rotating dislocations are displaced.

Although this is a somewhat ideal model, dislocation generation at local regions of stress concentration is common. A simple example for a carbide inclusion in iron is shown in Fig. 8.4. When the precipitate has a complex shape the associated strain field and resultant dislocation distribution is correspondingly more complex and tangled arrays of dislocations are produced. Other stress concentrators such as surface irregularities, cracks, etc., have a similar effect.

## 8.5 Multiplication of Dislocations by Frank–Read Sources

To account for the large plastic strain that can be produced in crystals, it is necessary to have *regenerative multiplication* of dislocations. Two mechanisms are important. One is the *Frank–Read type sources* to be described in this section and the other is *multiple cross glide* described in section 8.6.

The first model proposed by Frank and Read resembles the model proposed to account for the role of dislocations in crystal growth. In an irregular array some dislocations lie partly in their slip planes and partly in other planes. This is illustrated in Fig. 8.5(a). The length *BC* of the edge dislocation *ABC* lies in the slip plane *CEF* and can move freely in this plane. The length *AB* is not in the slip plane and is sessile. Thus *BC* will be anchored at one end and can only move by rotating about *B*. The dislocation will tend to wind up into a spiral as illustrated in Fig. 8.5(b). Two things are noted about this mechanism:

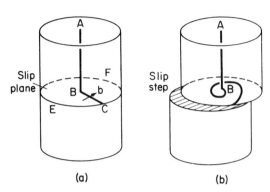

(a)                                    (b)

FIG. 8.5. Single ended Frank-Read source. (a) Dislocation lying partly in slip plane *CEF*. (b) Formation of a slip step and spiral dislocation by rotation of *BC* about *B*.

(a) Each revolution around *B* produces a displacement of the crystal above the slip plane by one atom spacing *b*; the process is *regenerative* since the process can repeat itself so that *n* revolutions will produce a displacement *nb*. A large *slip step* will be produced at the surface of the crystal.

(b) The spiralling around *B* results in an increase in the total length of dislocation line. This mechanism is similar to the single ended sources mentioned in section 7.4.

The well-known *Frank–Read source* is an extension of the above mechanism to a dislocation line held at each end as illustrated in Fig. 8.6. The dislocation line *DD'* lies in a slip plane represented by the plane of the paper. It is held at both ends by an unspecified barrier, which may be dislocation intersections or nodes, composite jogs, precipitates, etc. An applied stress $\tau$ tends to make the dislocation bow out as described in section 4.4, and the radius of curvature $\varrho$ depends on the stress according to equation (4.19). As the dislocation bows out under an increasing stress a minimum value of $\varrho$ is reached at the position illustrated in Fig. 8.6(b). The radius of curvature will be $L/2$, where $L$ is the length of *DD'*. For $\tau \geqslant Gb/L$, taking $\alpha = 0.5$, the dislocation will continue to expand under a

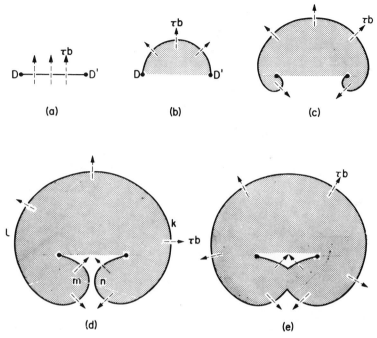

FIG. 8.6. Diagrammatic representation of the dislocation movement in the Frank-Read source. Unit slip has occurred in the shaded area. (From READ (1953), *Dislocations in Crystals*, McGraw-Hill.)

decreasing stress. The subsequent events are shown in Fig. 8.6(c–e); the dislocation forms a large kidney-shaped loop and when the segments at *m* and *n* meet they will annihilate each other to form a large loop and a new dislocation *DD'*. This can be visualised by considering *DD'* to be in a screw orientation. At sites *k* and *l* in Fig. 8.6(d) the dislocation is in positive and negative edge orientations respectively because the dislocation line is normal to the vector. Similarly, at *m* and *n* the dislocation will be in positive and negative edge orientation and, since they have a mutual attraction (section 4.6), they will combine and annihilate at this point. The process is *regenerative* and a series of loops can be produced. An excellent example of a Frank–Read source is illustrated in Fig. 8.7. The dislocation is held at each end by other parts of the dislocation network. These are not is the plane of the loops and are consequently out of focus. The dislocation lines tend to lie along specific directions in which they have a minimum energy indicating the strong anisotropy of this material.

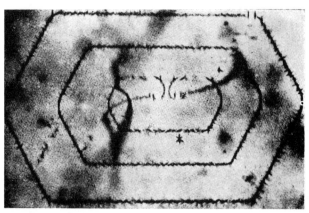

FIG. 8.7. Frank-Read source in a silicon crystal. The dislocations have been revealed by the decoration technique described in section 2.3. (From DASH (1957), *Dislocation and Mechanical Properties of Crystals*, Wiley.)

Considerable multiplication probably occurs by the Frank–Read mechanism, but additional processes must occur to account for the experimental observations. For example, the Frank–Read source does not explain the broadening of slip bands which is a common feature of the early stages of deformation of some crystals, e.g. iron and lithium fluoride.

### 8.6 Multiplication by Multiple Cross Glide

An example of the multiplication of dislocations associated with the initiation and broadening of a slip band is shown in Fig. 8.8, from work by Gilman and Johnston on lithium fluoride. The dislocations are revealed by the etch pit technique (section 2.2); a succession of etching and deformation treatments revealed the growth of the slip band. Initially (Fig. 8.8(a)), the slip band started as a

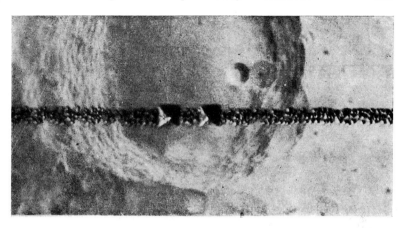

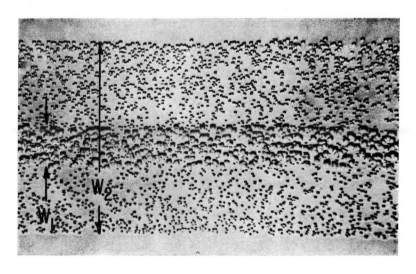

FIG. 8.8. Lateral growth of glide bands in lithium fluoride. (a) Glide band formed at a single loop. Large pits show the position of the loop. Small pits show that new dislocations lie on both sides of the glide plane of the original loop. (b) Widening of a glide band. (From GILMAN and JOHNSTON, *Solid State Physics*, **13**, 147, 1962.)

single loop of dislocation and the two points of emergence are revealed by the two large pits. Deformation resulted in the formation of dislocations on each side of the original loop. Since the band of dislocation etch pits has a finite width, it follows that the dislocations do not lie on the same glide plane, but on a set of parallel glide planes. Widening of a glide band is shown in Fig. 8.8(b); after the first deformation the band was $W_1$ wide and after the second deformation $W_2$ wide. The dislocation density is approximately uniform throughout the band.

The widening can be accounted for by a process called *multiple cross glide*. In principle, it is the same as the process illustrated in Fig. 3.7. Thus, a screw dislocation lying along $AB$ can cross glide onto position $CD$ on a parallel glide plane. If the stress is greater on the primary plane the composite jogs $AC$ and $BD$ are relatively immobile. However the segments lying in the primary slip planes will be free to expand and can each operate as a Frank–Read source. When cross glide can occur readily, the Frank–Read sources may never complete a cycle and there will be one continonus dislocation line lying on each of many parallel glide planes, connected by jogs. Thus, it is possible for a single dislocation loop to expand and multiply in such a way that the slip spreads from plane to plane, so producing a wide slip band. Multiple cross glide is a more effective mechanism than the simple Frank–Read source since it results in a more rapid multiplication.

### 8.7 Multiplication from Prismatic Loops

Many examples have been described of the formation of prismatic loops during quenching, irradiation and plastic deformation. The loops observed normally have diameters in the range 20–100 nm and they can be produced in large numbers. Any process which enlarges the loops is essentially dislocation multiplication.

A prismatic loop can glide only on the prismatic surface containing the dislocation line and its Burgers vector. However, if the Burgers vector is not a common slip vector, as for example in the Frank sessile dislocation loop in a face-centred cubic lattice, no dislocation multiplication will occur by glide. When the loop Burgers vector is a slip vector an applied stress will cause the loop to move. In Fig. 8.1 the prismatic loops have been pushed along the glide cylinder by interaction between successive loops but there is no increase in the dislocation line length of individual loops. However, under an externally applied shear stress different segments of the loop will tend to move in opposite directions. Consider the square loop in Fig. 8.9(a)

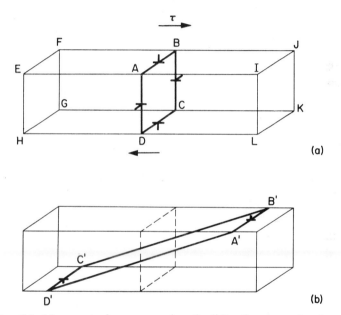

FIG. 8.9. Movement of a square prismatic dislocation loop due to an externally applied stress.

formed by the collapse of a vacancy platelet. The edge dislocation segments *AB* and *CD* have the same Burgers vectors (they are part of the same dislocation line), but they have opposite senses. The applied shear stress causes *AB* to move in one direction and *CD* in the opposite direction. The segments *BC* and *DA* are unaffected by the applied stress but as *AB* and *CD* bow out in their slip planes they will drag *BC* and $DA$ into the position illustrated in Fig. 8.9(b). A large increase in the length of the dislocation line is produced. The stress required for this process will increase with decreasing loop size.

## 8.8 Multiplication by Climb

Two mechanisms, involving climb, which increase the total dislocation length, have been described already; (a) the expansion of a prismatic loop and (b) the spiralling of a dislocation with a predominantly screw character (section 3,7). A *regenerative multiplication* known as the *Bardeen–Herring source* can occur by climb in a similar way to the Frank–Read mechanism illustrated in Fig. 8.6. Suppose that the dislocation line $DD'$ in Fig. 8.6 is an edge dislocation with the extra half plane in the plane of the paper above $DD'$. If the dislocation line is held at $D$ and $D'$ the presence of an excess concentration of vacancies will cause the dislocation to climb. An additional condition to the normal Frank–Read source must be satisfied if this process is to be regenerative; the anchor points $D$ and $D'$ must end on screw dislocations. If this were not so, one cycle of the source, Fig. 8.6(d), would remove the extra half plane without creating a new dislocation along $DD'$. Bardeen–Herring sources have been observed experimentally as illustrated in Fig. 8.10 for an aluminium–3·5 per cent magnesium alloy quenched from 550°C into silicone oil. The large concentration of excess vacancies has resulted in the formation of four concentric loops. Each loop represents the removal of a plane of atoms. More complicated source arrangements have also been observed in this alloy (Westmacott *et al.*, 1962).

Before a dislocation will bow out by climb due to the diffusion of vacancies or interstitial atoms it is necessary that the gain in energy, due to the loss or creation of defects, is larger than the change in energy of the dislocation line. This is analogous to the slip problem (section 4.5) in which the stress to bow out a dislocation is given by equation (4.19). The work done by a stress $\tau$ in moving a unit length of dislocation line a distance $dx$ is $\tau b\, dx$ per unit length of line. The

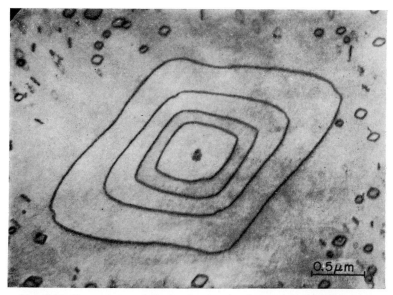

FIG. 8.10. Transmission electron micrograph of concentric loops formed at a climb source in aluminium 3·5 per cent magnesium alloy quenched from 550°C. (From WESTMACOTT, BARNES and SMALLMAN, *Phil. Mag.* 7, 1585, 1962.)

corresponding energy required to create sufficient vacancies to move the dislocation the same distance will be the energy to form a vacancy $U_v$ multiplied by the number of vacancies per unit length, $b\,dx/\Omega_0$, where $\Omega_0$ is the atomic volume. Equating the two expressions

$$\tau b\,dx = \frac{U_v b\,dx}{\Omega_0},$$

therefore

$$\tau = \frac{U_v}{\Omega_0}. \tag{8.9}$$

The condition for a dislocation to bow out is obtained by substituting for $\tau$ in equation (4.19),

$$U_v > \frac{\alpha G b \Omega_0}{\varrho}. \tag{8.10}$$

If a crystal contains $n$ vacant sites, and $n_{eq}$ is the equilibrium number of vacant sites, then

$$U_v = kT \ln \left( \frac{n}{n_{eq}} \right) \tag{8.11}$$

Substituting in relation (8.10) gives

$$\ln \left( \frac{n}{n_{eq}} \right) > \frac{\alpha G b \Omega_0}{\varrho k T} . \tag{8.12}$$

Taking $G = 50 \, \text{GN m}^{-2}$, $b = 0.2 \, \text{nm}$, $\Omega_0 = 0.01 \, \text{nm}^3$, $k = 1.38 \times 10^{-23} \, \text{JK}^{-1}$, $T = 1000 \, \text{K}$, $2\varrho = 1 \, \mu\text{m}$ gives

$$\ln \left( \frac{n}{n_{eq}} \right) > 10^{-2}, \tag{8.13}$$

$$\frac{n}{n_{eq}} = e^{0.01} = 1.01.$$

Thus a departure from the normal equilibrium concentration of the order of only one part in a hundred is sufficient to cause a dislocation line of length 1 $\mu$m to act as a source of dislocation rings.

## Further Reading

ASHBY, M. F. and JOHNSON, L. (1969) "On the generation of dislocations at misfitting particles in a ductile matrix", *Phil Mag.* **20,** 1009.

BARDEEN, J. and HERRING, C. (1952) "Diffusion in alloys and the Kirkendall effect", *Imperfections in Nearly Perfect Crystals*, p. 261, Wiley.

BROWN, L. M. and WOODHOUSE, G. R. (1970) "The loss of coherency of precipitates and the generation of dislocations", *Phil. Mag.* **21,** 329.

COTTRELL, A. H. and BILBY, B. A. (1951) "Growth of deformation twins", *Phil. Mag.* **42,** 573.

DASH, W. C. (1957) "Observation of dislocations in silicon", *Dislocations and the Mechanical Properties of Crystals*, p. 57, Wiley.

DOREMUS, R. H., ROBERTS, B. W. and TURNBULL, D. (Eds.) (1958) *Growth and Perfection of Crystals*, Wiley. This book contains a number of interesting papers on crystal growth and whiskers including:

NABARRO, F. R. N. and JACKSON, P. J. "Growth of crystal whiskers", p. 11.

BRENNER, S. S. "Properties of whiskers", p. 157.

CHALMERS, B. "Growth of crystals of pure materials", p. 291.

DASH, W. C. "Growth of silicon crystals free from dislocations", p. 361.
CABRERA, N. and VERMILYEA, D. A. "Growth of crystals from solution", p. 393.
ELBAUM, C. (1959) "Substructure in crystals grown from the melt", *Progress in Metal Physics*, Vol. 8, p. 203, Pergamon, London.
FRANK, F. C. (1949) "Crystal growth", *Disc. Faraday Soc.* **5**, 1.
FRANK, F. C. (1952) "Crystal growth and dislocations", *Adv. Physics*, **1**, 91.
GILMAN, J. J. (1959) "Dislocation sources in crystals", *J. Appl. Phys.* **30**, 1584.
GILMAN, J. J. and JOHNSTON, W. G. (1957) "Origin and growth of glide bands", *Dislocations and Mechanical Properties of Crystals*, p. 116, Wiley.
GILMAN, J. J. and JOHNSTON, W. G. (1962) "Dislocations in lithium fluoride", *Solid State Physics*, **13**, 147.
JONES, D. A. and MITCHELL, J. W. (1958) "Observation of helical dislocations in silver chloride", *Phil. Mag.* **3**, 1.
KUHLMANN-WILSDORF, D. (1958) "Origin of dislocations", *Phil. Mag.* **3**, 125.
REID, C. N., GILBERT, A. and ROSENFIELD, A. R. (1965) "Dislocation multiplication" *Phil. Mag.* **12**, 409.
VERMA, A. R. (1953) *Crystal Growth and Dislocations*, Butterworth, London.
WESTMACOTT, K. H., BARNES, R. S. and SMALLMAN, R. E. (1962) "Observation of a dislocation climb source", *Phil. Mag.* **7**, 1585.

CHAPTER 9

# Dislocation Arrays and Crystal Boundaries

## 9.1 Plastic Deformation, Recovery and Recrystallisation

Plastic deformation of crystalline materials leads to the formation of three-dimensional arrays or distributions of dislocations which are characteristic of (1) crystal structure of the material being deformed, (2) temperature of deformation, (3) strain, and (4) strain rate. Additionally, such features as grain boundaries, precipitates, and stacking fault energy affect the distribution of the dislocations. Two distributions are illustrated in Fig. 9.1, which shows the effect of deforming pure iron specimens at 20°C and −135°C, respectively. Deformation at 20°C has resulted in the formation of dense *tangles of dislocations* arranged in *walls* surrounding regions or *cells* almost free from dislocations. The *cell size* reaches a limit in the early stages of deformation and changes only slightly thereafter. The cell walls tend to orient themselves in certain crystallographic directions. Deformation at −135°C produces a much more homogeneous distribution of dislocations.

The hardening of crystals during plastic deformation is due to the increase in dislocation density and the mutual interaction between dislocations (Chapter 10). The introduction of dislocations produces a large increase in the elastic strain energy of the crystal *(stored*

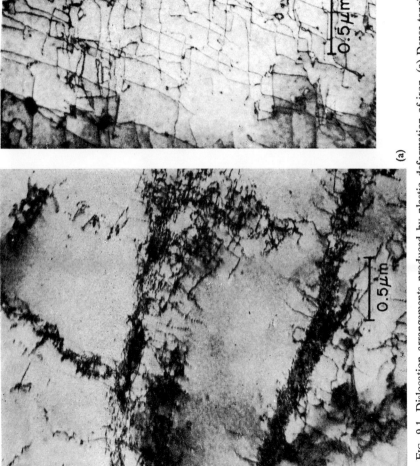

FIG. 9.1. Dislocation arrangements produced by plastic deformation of iron. (a) Dense tangles and dislocation free cells formed after 9 per cent strain at 20°C. (b) Uniform array of straight dislocations formed after 7 per cent strain at −135°C. (From KEH and WEISSMANN (1963), *Electron Microscopy and Strength of Crystals*, p. 231, Interscience.)

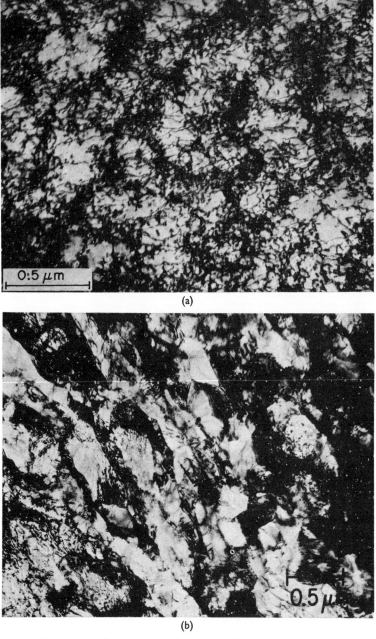

(a)

(b)

Fig. 9.2. Transmission electron micrographs illustrating the structure of deformed and annealed 3·25 per cent silicon iron. (a) Approximately uniform distribution of dislocations in a crystal rolled 20 per cent. (b) Formation of small sub-grains in rolled material annealed 15 min at 500°C. (c) As for (b) annealed 15 min at 600°C. (d) As for (b) annealed 30 min at 600°C. (From Hu, *Trans Met. Soc. A.I.M.E.* **230**, 572, 1964.)

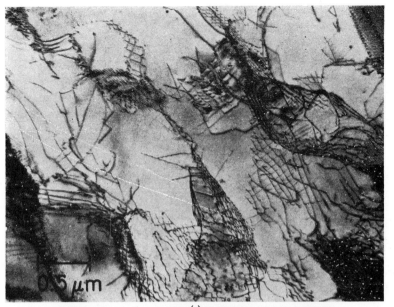

(c)

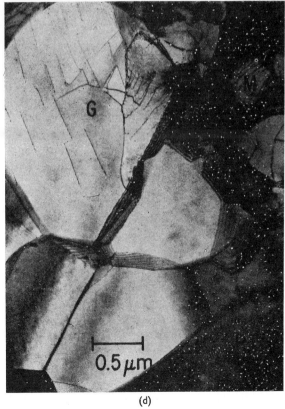

(d)

*energy)* which will be released if the dislocations either annihilate each other by mutual interactions or rearrange themselves into low energy configurations. Additional energy will be stored in the crystal if point defects are produced during deformation. The low-energy stable configurations are called *low-angle boundaries* and can be represented by a uniform array of one, two, three or more sets of dislocations (sections 9.2 and 9.3). They separate regions of the crystal which differ in orientation by $<5°$. A considerable amount of energy is released by the local rearrangement of the dislocations in the *tangles* and further release of energy occurs when low-angle boundaries are formed. Both these processes involve climb of the dislocations and will occur, therefore, only when there is sufficient thermal activation to allow local and long-range diffusion of point defects. These changes are accompanied by a pronounced softening of the dislocation hardened crystal. The process is called *recovery* and it occurs when a plastically deformed crystal is heated to moderate temperatures. The later stages of the recovery process in which low-angle boundaries are formed is called *polygonisation.*

When a heavily cold worked metal is heated above a critical temperature new grains relatively free from dislocations are produced in the "recovered" structure, resulting in a process called *recrystallisation.* Large angle grain boundaries with a misorientation $>10°$ are produced. The sequence of photographs in Fig. 9.2 illustrates the change from a heavily deformed structure with a uniform distribution of tangled dislocations to a recrystallised structure containing large and small angle grain boundaries. The grain structure is small immediately after recrystallisation but grows progressively with longer annealing times and higher temperatures. This is called *grain growth* and results in a small reduction in energy because the total area of grain boundary is reduced.

The basic process in the formation of low-angle boundaries is illustrated in its most simple form in Fig. 9.3. Consider a crystal which is bent about the $x$-axis; the dislocations will be distributed randomly on the glide planes in the way illustrated in Fig. 9.3(a). The energy of the crystal can be reduced by rearranging the dis-

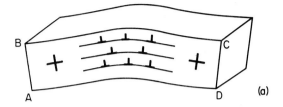

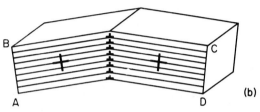

FIG. 9.3. Formation of a low angle boundary. (a) Bent crystal with random dislocations. (b) Rearrangement of dislocations to form symmetrical tilt boundary. Both climb and glide are required to produce this boundary.

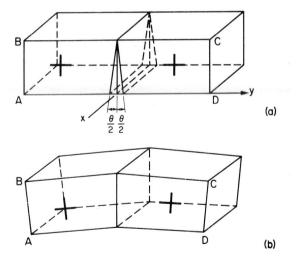

FIG. 9.4. Geometry of the formation of a symmetrical tilt boundary. The relative rotation of the two crystals is produced by cutting a wedge from the perfect crystal.

locations into a vertical wall to form a symmetrical tilt boundary, Fig. 9.3(b) (section 9.2). Alternatively, imagine that a thin wedge-shaped section, symmetrical about the plane $y = 0$, is cut from the perfect crystal *ABCD*, Fig. 9.4(a), and that the two cut faces are

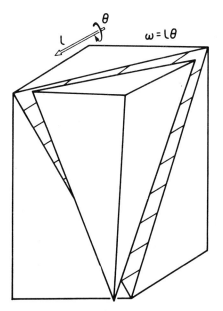

FIG. 9.5. Formation of a general grain boundary with 5 degrees of freedom. (From READ (1953), *Dislocations in Crystals*, McGraw-Hill.)

then placed together as in Fig. 9.4(b). This is geometrically the same as the tilt boundaries in Fig. 9.3(c) and illustrates an important feature of small angle boundaries, namely that they have *no long range stress field*. The strain is localised in the region around the dislocations.

The example illustrated in Fig. 9.4 is a boundary with *one degree of freedom* since the axis of relative rotation is a cube axis and the boundary is symmetrically placed with respect to the two grains. In the general case illustrated in Fig. 9.5, the wedge is produced by cutting the crystal along two arbitrary planes and placing the grains together with a twist. The orientations of the two cuts and the magnitude of the twist define *5 degrees of freedom;* three due to the relative rotation of the adjoining crystals about three perpendicular axes and two due to the orientation of the boundary with respect to the crystals.

The requirement that there are no long-range stress fields places severe conditions on the dislocation geometry of low angle boundaries and this is discussed in sections 9.3 and 9.4. The regular dislocation

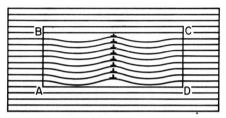

FIG. 9.6. Representation of the long-range stress fields of a dislocation boundary.

arrays observed after recovery are true low angle boundaries. These boundaries are not likely to be formed during plastic deformation because the boundaries formed by deformation have long-range stress fields even though they may consist of simple dislocation arrangements. There are no external constraints on the two grains illustrated in Figs. 9.3 and 9.4. If, however, the same boundary was formed by plastically deforming the two crystals to the required shape instead of by removing wedge-shaped sections, the material surrounding the boundary would produce constraints which represent a long range stress field. The nature of the long-range stress fields is illustrated diagrammatically in Fig. 9.6 in which a tilt boundary is surrounded completely by an underformed crystal. The tangle boundaries in Fig. 9.1 may well be of this type.

## 9.2 Simple Dislocation Boundaries

The simplest boundary is the *symmetrical tilt boundary* (Figs. 2.3 and 9.4). In a simple cubic lattice with edge dislocations **b** = [010], the boundary will consist of a sheet of equally spaced dis-

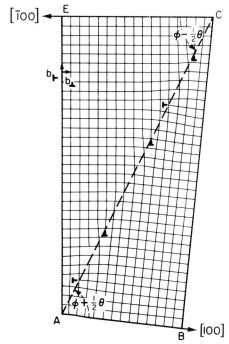

Fig. 9.7. Tilt boundary with two degrees of freedom. This is the same boundary as in Fig. 9.3 except that the plane of the boundary makes an arbitrary angle $\phi$ with the mean of the (010) planes in the two grains. The atom planes end on the boundary in two sets of evenly spaced edge dislocations. (From READ (1953), *Dislocations in Crystals*, McGraw-Hill.)

locations lying parallel to the *x*-axis; the plane of the sheet will be the symmetry plane $y = 0$, i.e. (010). The crystals on each side of the boundary are rotated by equal and opposite amounts about the *x*-axis and differ in orientation by the angle $\theta$ (Fig. 2.3). If the spacing of the dislocations is $D$, then:

$$\frac{b}{D} = 2 \sin \frac{\theta}{2} \qquad (9.1)$$

and for small values of $\theta$ (in radians)

$$\frac{b}{D} \sim \theta. \qquad (9.2)$$

If $\theta = 1°$ and $b = 0.25$ nm the spacing between dislocations will be 14 nm. When the spacing is less than a few lattice spacings, say five, $\theta \sim 10°$ and the individual identity of the dislocations is in doubt, the boundary is called a *large-angle boundary*. Experimental evidence for tilt boundaries has been presented in Fig. 2.3. Many such observations of boundaries have been reported using decoration and thin film transmission electron microscope techniques.

A *more general tilt boundary* is illustrated in Fig. 9.7. By introducing a second degree of freedom the boundary plane can be rotated about the x-axis. The boundary plane is no longer a symmetry plane for the two crystals but forms an angle $\phi$ with the plane of symmetry. Two sets of atom planes end on the boundary and the geometrical conditions require the boundary to consist of two sets of uniformly spaced edge dislocations with mutually perpendicular Burgers vectors, $b_1$ and $b_2$. The spacing of the two sets are, respectively:

$$D_1 = \frac{b_1}{\theta \sin \phi},$$
$$D_2 = \frac{b_2}{\theta \cos \phi}, \qquad (9.3)$$

providing $\theta$ is small.

A simple boundary formed from a *cross grid of pure screw dislocations* is illustrated in Fig. 9.8. A single set of screw dislocations has a long range stress field and is therefore unstable but the stress field is cancelled by the second set of screw dislocations. The two sets of equally spaced parallel dislocations lie in the boundary which also lies in the plane of the diagram. They produce a rotation about

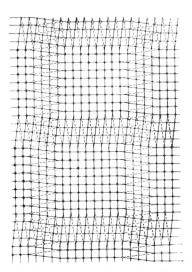

FIG. 9.8. A pure twist boundary parallel to the plane of the figure. The two grains have a small relative rotation about their cube axis, which is normal to the boundary. The open circles represent atoms just above the boundary and the solid circles atoms just below. The atoms join continuously except along the two sets of screw dislocations, which form a cross grid. (From READ (1953), *Dislocations in Crystals*, McGraw-Hill.)

an axis normal to the boundary of one-half of the crystal with respect to the other. Such a boundary is called a *twist boundary*. The spacing between dislocations in each set is:

$$D = \frac{b}{\theta}.$$

### 9.3 General Low-angle Boundaries

Following Read (1953) the *5 degrees of freedom* of a grain boundary can be represented by (a) the magnitude of the relative rotation $\theta$ that would bring the grains into perfect registry, (b) the axis of relative rotation, and (c) the orientation of the boundary. If $\mathbf{l}$ is a unit vector parallel to the axis of relative rotation, the rotation of one grain relative to the other is a vector $\mathbf{w} = \mathbf{l}\theta$ (see Fig. 9.5). The three components of **w** along the three crystal axes represent three degrees of freedom of the relative rotation. The orientation of the boundary can also be specified by a unit vector **n** normal to the plane of the boundary. The tilt and twist boundaries can now be defined as follows: in a tilt boundary, **l** and **n** are at right-angles and in a twist boundary **l** = **n**. In the examples in section 9.2 the tilt boundaries are described by arrays of edge dislocations and the twist boundaries by screw dislocations. In the general case both edge and screw components are required in a boundary, and any given boundary will have a mixed *tilt* and *twist* character.

The orientation of the crystals and the boundary formed in the way illustrated in Figs. 9.4 and 9.5 can be defined by the parameters **l**, **n** and $\theta$. Frank (1950) has derived a relation which may be used to determine the arrangements of dislocations which will produce such a boundary, or conversely the orientation of a boundary produced by a given set of dislocations or *dislocation network*. For a general boundary, Frank's relation is

or

$$\mathbf{d} = (\mathbf{r} \times \mathbf{l}) \, 2 \sin \frac{\theta}{2}$$

$$\mathbf{d} = (\mathbf{r} \times \mathbf{l}) \, \theta \tag{9.4}$$

for small values of $\theta$. The vector **r** represents an arbitrary straight line lying in the plane of the boundary which contains the dislocation network, and **d** is the sum of the Burgers vectors of all the dislocations intersected by **r**. A number of facts should be noted regarding the application of this relation:

(a) It applies only to boundaries which are essentially flat and have no long-range stress field, i.e. the elastic distortion is restricted to the region close to the dislocations.

(b) The formula does not uniquely determine the dislocations present, or their pattern, for a given orientation of crystal and boundary. Thus, a variety of possibilities may arise and the most probable will be the one of lowest energy.

(c) The density of a given set of dislocations in a boundary is directly proportional to $\theta$ (for small $\theta$).

(d) Each set of dislocation lines will be straight, equally spaced and parallel even for a boundary containing several sets of dislocations with different Burgers vectors.

The application of the Frank relation will be illustrated by two simple examples: firstly, the determination of the dislocation arrangement in a boundary when $\theta$, $\mathbf{l}$ and $\mathbf{n}$ are known, and secondly, the determination of the orientation of a net from a given dislocation arrangement.

Firstly, consider a boundary in a simple cubic lattice such that $\mathbf{l} = [001]$ and $\mathbf{n} = [100]$. Take $\mathbf{r}$ lines in this boundary and determine the corresponding values of $\mathbf{d}$. Using Frank's equation, when $\mathbf{r}$ is a unit vector in the [001] direction

$$\mathbf{d} = [001] \times [001] \, 2 \sin \frac{\theta}{2} = 0. \tag{9.5}$$

The simplest case for $\mathbf{d} = 0$ is when $\mathbf{r}$ does not cut any dislocations so that all the dislocations must lie parallel to [001]. When $\mathbf{r}$ is a unit vector in the [010] direction

$$\mathbf{d} = [010] \times [001] \, 2 \sin \frac{\theta}{2} = [100] \, 2 \sin \frac{\theta}{2} \simeq [100] \, \theta. \tag{9.6}$$

This equation can be written in terms of the expected dislocations in the simple cubic lattice, i.e. dislocations of the type $\langle 100 \rangle$; if $\mathbf{b} = [100]$

$$\mathbf{d} = \frac{\theta \mathbf{b}}{b}. \tag{9.7}$$

This corresponds to a set of dislocations with Burgers vector $\mathbf{b}$ and spacing $D = b/\theta$. Thus the simplest dislocation arrangement for the boundary is a single set of equally spaced dislocations, Burgers vector $\mathbf{b}$, lying parallel to [001]. This is the arrangement of dislocations illustrated in Fig. 2.3.

Secondly, following Frank (1955), consider a dislocation network in a face-centred cubic lattice. The dislocations can be described using the Thompson notation (section 5.4). Suppose that the dislocations form a regular hexagonal pattern as illustrated in Fig. 9.9. The plane of the net and the Burgers vectors of the dislocations are co-planar, $\mathbf{AB} = \frac{1}{2}[\bar{1}10]$, $\mathbf{BC} = \frac{1}{2}[10\bar{1}]$, and $\mathbf{CA} = \frac{1}{2}[0\bar{1}1]$. It is important that the sequence of lettering around any node is consistent. The Burgers vector of each dislocation is represented by two letters written on either side of it. The lettering should be such that any track around the node

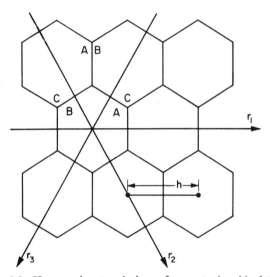

Fig. 9.9. Hexagonal network in a face-centred cubic lattice.

makes a continuous path, for example, *AB, BC, CA*, or *AB, CA, BC*, but not *BC, CA, BA*, or *AB, BC, CD*. Given that *h* is the distance between the centres of the mesh, the orientation of the plane of the net and the individual dislocations in the net can now be determined. If an **r** line is placed horizontally on the net in Fig. 9.9, i.e. $\mathbf{r}_1$, it crosses $|\mathbf{r}_1|/h$ dislocations of Burgers vector **AB**. The number of dislocations crossed is $\mathbf{d}/\mathbf{AB}$. Thus,

$$\frac{\mathbf{d}}{|\mathbf{r}_1|} = \frac{(\mathbf{AB})}{h}. \tag{9.8}$$

Similarly for the other **r** lines taken at 120° to the first one, i.e. $\mathbf{r}_2$

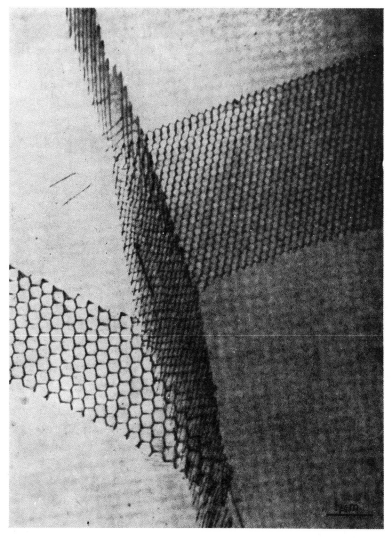

FIG. 9.10. Transmission electron micrograph of extensive dislocation networks in body-centred cubic iron. Each networks consist of three sets of dislocations, Burgers vectors $\frac{1}{2}\langle 111 \rangle$, $\frac{1}{2}\langle 111 \rangle$ and $\langle 100 \rangle$. The plane of the networks is almost parallel to the plane of the foil (courtesy DADIAN and TALBOT–BESNARD).

and $\mathbf{r}_3$, $\mathbf{d}/|\mathbf{r}_2| = (\mathbf{BC})/h$ and $\mathbf{d}/|\mathbf{r}_3| = (\mathbf{CA})/h$ respectively. It follows from the geometry of the net that $|\mathbf{d}|/|\mathbf{r}|$ has the same value for the three intersecting directions of $\mathbf{r}$. This can only be true if $\mathbf{l}$ is normal to the plane of the net, and, moreover, $\mathbf{l}$ must be normal to $\mathbf{AB}$, $\mathbf{BC}$, and $\mathbf{CA}$. Hence the arrangement of dislocations represents a twist boundary on the (111) plane, with the angle of rotation:

$$\theta = 2\sin^{-1}\left(\frac{b}{2h}\right) \simeq \left(\frac{b}{h}\right) \tag{9.9}$$

where $b$ is the elementary Burgers vector length $|\mathbf{AB}|$. Such a net of regular hexagons cannot lie in any other plane without producing long range stress fields in the crystal. Any deviation from the (111) boundary plane must be accompanied by a modification of the regular hexagon structure if long-range stresses are to be avoided. The character of the dislocations in the network can be found since each of the $\mathbf{r}$ lines chosen cuts only one set of dislocations. From Frank's equation, their Burgers vectors must be normal to $\mathbf{r}$ and $\mathbf{l}$, and therefore they are parallel to the dislocations, since the $\mathbf{r}$ lines cut the dislocations at right angles. All the dislocations in the net are pure screws, lying along $[\bar{1}10]$, $[10\bar{1}]$ and $[0\bar{1}1]$. The arrangement of dislocations in a typical boundary in a body-centred cubic structure is shown in Fig. 9.10.

Although low-angle boundaries are formed primarily under conditions in which dislocations can climb freely, it is possible to produce them by slip, but the geometrical conditions are very restrictive. The orientation and character of the dislocations in the boundary must have common slip Burgers vectors and lie on slip planes, and also satisfy the Frank equation.

## 9.4 Stress Field of Dislocation Arrays

The simple arguments in section 9.1 show that a dislocation array may have both long and short range stress fields. The distribution of stress is sensitive to the arrangement, orientation, and Burgers vectors of the dislocations composing the boundary. A few examples of the most elementary boundaries are sufficient to illustrate these points.

The components of the stress field of single edge and screw dislocations have been given in equations (4.6) and (4.5), respectively. The total stress field of an array is obtained by a summation of the components of the stress field of the individual dislocations sited in the array. Thus, consider a wall of edge dislocations making up a symmetrical tilt boundary lying in the plane $x = 0$ with the dislocations parallel to the $z$-axis. The stress field of this boundary is given by

$$\sigma_x = -\frac{Gb}{2\pi(1-\nu)} \sum_{n=1}^{N} \frac{y_n(3x^2+y_n^2)}{(x^2+y_n^2)^2}, \qquad (9.10)$$

$$\sigma_y = \frac{Gb}{2\pi(1-\nu)} \sum_{n=1}^{N} \frac{y_n(x^2-y_n^2)}{(x^2+y_n^2)^2}, \qquad (9.11)$$

$$\tau_{xy} = \frac{Gb}{2\pi(1-\nu)} \sum_{n=1}^{N} \frac{x(x^2-y_n^2)}{(x^2+y_n^2)^2}, \qquad (9.12)$$

etc. where $N$ is the total number of dislocations in the wall, $b$ is the magnitude of the Burgers vectors of the individual dislocations, $y_n = y+nD$, and $D$ is the spacing of the dislocations. It will be noted that when $N = 1$ these equations are identical to equations (4.6). The summation can be illustrated by a simple graphical approach. Figure 9.11 represents the stress field, component $\sigma_z$, around a single edge dislocation as given by equation (4.6). The stress field of a two dislocation wall, spacing $D$, is obtained by superimposing the two stress fields, distance $D$ apart and adding the components as in Fig. 9.12. There is a considerable cancellation of the stress fields between the two dislocations and the total strain energy of the two dislocations so arranged is smaller than if the dislocations were separate. Graphical summation is difficult when there are many dislocations in the wall. Mathematical summation of equations (9.10)–(9.12) is difficult also, and precise solutions have been obtained only for infinite arrays of dislocations (Li, 1963). One such solution is plotted graphically in Fig. 9.13 for the shear stress field $\tau_{xy}$. This diagram illustrates a number of important features of an *infinite wall of edge dislocations* which are common to

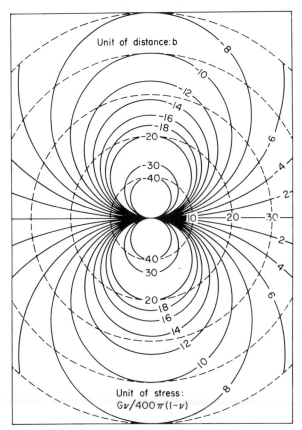

FIG. 9.11. The stress field of a single edge dislocation, $\sigma_z$. (From Li (1963), *Electron Microscopy and Strength of Crystals*, p. 713. Interscience.)

all low angle boundaries. The periodic stress field of the equally spaced dislocations results in a cancellation of the long range stress fields of the single dislocations such that $\tau_{xy}$ is negligible at distances greater than $\pm D$ from the boundary. Because the stress fields are localised at the boundary the strain energy will be small and therefore the boundary represents a stable configuration with respect to slip. However, the dislocations in the boundary can climb resulting in an increased separation of the dislocations and a reduction in $\theta$.

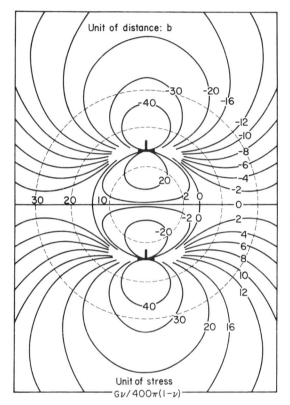

FIG. 9.12. The stress field of a vertical wall of two edge dislocations spaced 28$b$ apart, $\sigma_z$.

If the dislocations in the vertical wall were to be moved by slip so that the boundary made an angle $\phi$ with the original low-energy position, it can be shown that the wall will have a long-range stress field and a higher energy because the stress field of the individual dislocations no longer cancel each other so effectively. Such a boundary is most likely to be formed during plastic deformation. The long-range stresses can be removed by the boundary combining with a second wall of dislocations with Burgers vectors normal to the original ones as shown in the stable tilt boundary in Fig. 9.7. Similar arguments

(Li, 1963) can be used to show that an infinite wall of parallel screw dislocations always has a long-range stress field, which is removed by the introduction of a second set of screw dislocations to form a cross grid as in Fig. 9.8.

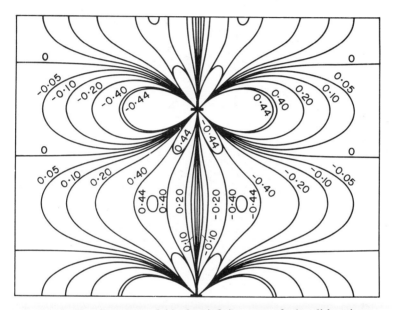

FIG. 9.13. The shear stress field of an infinite array of edge dislocations, $\tau_{xy}$. Unit of stress $Gb/2(1-v)D$. (From LI, *Acta Met.*, **8**, 296, 1960.)

Although infinite vertical edge dislocation walls have no long-range stresses a *finite wall* has and this has already been indicated in Figs. 9.6 and 9.12. No precise mathematical summation has been made for finite walls but approximate expressions have been derived (Li, 1963) which describe adequately the stress field except close to the dislocations.

As in the case of a single dislocation, work will be done when a dislocation is introduced into the stress field of a dislocation wall. The force required can be determined from equations of the type equation

(4.22), by introducing the appropriate values $\tau_{xy}$. The problem is complicated because of the movement of the boundary dislocations during interaction, and the different character of the interacting dislocation.

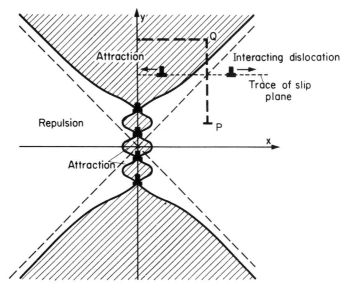

FIG. 9.14. Dislocation wall containing four like edge dislocations. Similar dislocations of the same sign in parallel glide planes are attracted or repelled depending on their position. The boundary between the shaded and unshaded regions is the line of zero shear stress.

Some qualitative features are worth noting and for simplicity a like-edge dislocation is considered to interact with a wall of edge dislocations. Depending on the length and orientation of the dislocation wall, interaction will occur over long and/or short distances from the boundary. The actual position of the slip plane of the edge dislocation, with respect to the boundary and the individual dislocations in the boundary, will affect the force. This is most clearly demonstrated by a consideration of the distribution of attractive and repulsive forces around the wall. Figure 9.13 shows that in some regions the shear stress field is negative and in others positive. In Fig. 9.14 the regions of attraction and repulsion around a finite vertical wall of edge dislocations are indicated. Apart from regions close to the wall of dislocations, attraction occurs only in the shaded regions above and below the wall. The magnitude of the attraction depends on the position of the dislocation and the spacing of the dislocations in the wall.

Figure 9.14 illustrates also a probable way in which a low-angle boundary develops during the *recovery process*. Dislocations in the unshaded regions will tend to be repelled by the boundary, but can climb by vacancy diffusion processes. If a dislocation at $P$ climbs into the shaded region it will then experience an attractive force tending to align the dislocation in the low-energy configuration at the top of the existing wall. The path taken is indicated by the dotted line.

### 9.5 Strain Energy of Dislocation Arrays

In principle the energy of a dislocation array can be calculated from the work done in producing the state of strain over the complete boundary. As in the case of a single dislocation the energy will be in two parts, elastic strain energy and core energy. The elastic strain energy of a symmetrical tilt boundary, i.e. an infinite vertical wall of edge dislocations, is equal to the total work done in forming the boundary which is equal to the sum of the work done in creating the individual dislocations. For the symmetrical tilt boundary this will be the same for each dislocation. The work done in introducing a single dislocation is obtained by integration of the shear stresses over the slip plane and multiplying by the relative displacement

$$E_1 = \frac{b}{2} \int_{r_0}^{\infty} \tau_{xy} \, dx. \tag{9.13}$$

The energy per unit area of boundary is found by multiplying by $\theta/b$, the number of dislocations per unit area. When the appropriate value of $\tau_{xy}$ is substituted in equation (9.13), the total elastic strain energy of the boundary can be written as

$$E = E_0 \theta (A - \ln \theta), \tag{9.14}$$

where

$$E_0 = \frac{Gb}{4\pi(1-\nu)},\qquad (9.15)$$

$$A = 1 + \ln\left(\frac{b}{2\pi r_0}\right).\qquad (9.16)$$

The energy of more complicated low-angle boundaries, such as a cross grid of screw dislocations, will include the interaction energy between sets of intersecting dislocations in addition to the self energy of the individual sets of dislocations. However, the energy per unit area can be expressed in the same form as equation (9.14). This expression contains two parts. Firstly, $E_0\theta A$, which represents the contribution to the total energy which is independent of the presence of other dislocations; the change with $\theta$ is directly proportional to the density of dislocations in the boundary. Since the core energy of a dislocation will be independent of other dislocations also, the equation can be adjusted to include the core energy by choosing a suitable value of $A$, and hence $r_0$, see equation (9.16). Secondly, $-E_0\theta \ln \theta$, which is the contribution arising from the mutual interaction of the stress fields of the dislocations in the boundary. The numerical increase in this term with increasing $\theta$ is consistent with the decrease in the long-range shear stresses with increasing $\theta$.

Experimental verification of equation (9.14) was one of the early successes of dislocation theory. The relative energy of a dislocation boundary was measured using the simple principle illustrated in Fig. 9.15. This shows three boundaries looking along the common axis of the grains. If $E_1$, $E_2$ and $E_3$ are the energies of the grain boundaries per unit area, which have the form given in equation (9.14), each boundary will have an effective surface tension equal to its energy. The situation will approximate, under equilibrium conditions to a triangle of forces, and for the equilibrium of these forces acting at a point

$$\frac{E_1}{\sin\psi_1} = \frac{E_2}{\sin\psi_2} = \frac{E_3}{\sin\psi_3}.\qquad (9.17)$$

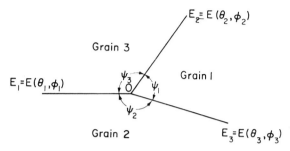

FIG. 9.15. Three grain boundaries that meet along a line (normal to the figure). Each boundary is defined by the angular misfit $\theta$ of the adjoining grains and the orientation $\phi$ of the boundary. (From READ (1953), *Dislocations in Crystals*, McGraw-Hill.)

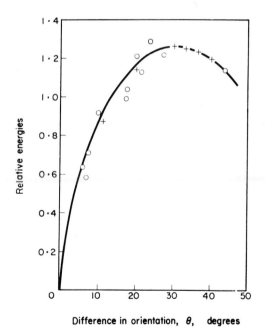

Difference in orientation, $\theta$, degrees

FIG. 9.16. Variation of the relative grain boundary energy with orientation for silicon iron tricrystals with a common [100] axis perpendicular to the plane of the specimen. The full line is the theoretical curve and the points experimental values of Dunn, Daniels and Bolton.

By measuring $\psi_1$, $\psi_2$ and $\psi_3$ and the misorientation across the boundaries it is possible to determine the relative energies. A typical set of results from work by Dunn and co-workers is shown in Fig. 9.16. The points represent the individual experimental observations and the full line represents the predicted variation of $E$ with $\theta$ using equation (9.14), and taking $A = 0.35$. The agreement is good even at large values of $\theta$, at which the dislocations in the boundary are very closely spaced and the theoretical equation has little real significance.

### 9.6 Movement of Boundaries

For the movement of a dislocation boundary three conditions must be satisfied. Firstly, the geometrical aspects governing the movement of individual dislocations. If slip is involved the boundary can move only when the dislocations in the boundary are free to move on the slip planes defined by the dislocation lines and their Burgers vectors. Secondly, the thermodynamic condition that movement results in either a reduction in the energy of the boundary or, in the case of movement induced by an externally applied stress, that the stress does work when the boundary moves. Thirdly, that the driving force due, for example, to the externally applied stress or the excess vacancy concentration is sufficient to produce dislocation movement. Some aspects of the stress required to move dislocations are considered in the next chapter.

The geometrical condition is particularly restrictive on the movement of simple dislocation boundaries and can be illustrated with reference to tilt boundaries which are required to move entirely by slip. The only *glissile* tilt boundary is one in which the dislocations have parallel glide planes. Consider the symmetrical tilt boundary illustrated in Fig. 9.17(a). A shear stress can be applied to the boundary by adding a weight to one end of the crystal as illustrated. For a shear stress $\tau$, acting on the slip planes in the slip direction, the force on every dislocation will be $b\tau$ per unit length, and since there are $\theta/b$ dislocation lines per unit surface, the force per unit surface on the boundary is

$$F = \theta\tau. \tag{9.18}$$

If this is sufficient to move the dislocations the boundary will move to the left as illustrated in Fig. 9.17(b). Since every dislocation remains in the same position relative to the other dislocations in the boundary the geometry of the boundary is conserved. The work done by $\tau$ is $\tau\theta$ per unit volume swept out by the boundary. The movement of such a boundary has been observed directly by Washburn and Parker (1952) in single crystals of zinc. Tilt boundaries were introduced by

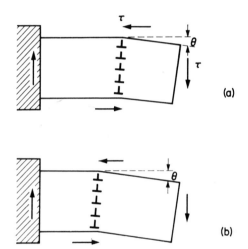

FIG. 9.17. Stress induced movement of a symmetrical pure tilt boundary.

bending the crystal, followed by an annealing treatment to produce polygonisation as in Fig. 9.3. The boundary was moved backwards and forwards by reversing the direction of the applied stress. It will be noted that the *semi-coherent twin boundary*, i.e. the moving dislocation boundary, illustrated in Fig. 6.8, is somewhat similar to the glissile tilt boundary in that all the dislocations have parallel Burgers vectors and glide planes; the boundary is highly mobile.

Now consider the tilt boundary illustrated in Fig. 9.7, in which the Burgers vector of the component edge dislocations are at right-angles. The movement of such a boundary under an applied stress has been considered by Shockley and Read (see Read, 1953). They describe three possibilities. (a) The dislocations move by pure glide and remain in the same plane parallel to the original boundary. This is possible only if one set of dislocations moves with the applied stress, and the other set against the applied stress. Since the slip planes are orthogonal the resolved shear stresses on the two systems are identical, and since the two sets of dislocations move equal distances the net work performed is zero. Thus, there will be no tendency for this to occur. (b) The dislocations move by pure glide but move in opposite directions. If both sets of dislocations move in such a way that work is done, the boundary will tend to split in the way illustrated in Fig. 9.18. However, the forces between dislocations will tend to keep the two boundaries together in the minimum energy configuration. Energy will be required and the process will be difficult. (c) The boundary moves uniformly as a whole, such that the dislocation arrangement in the boundary is conserved. This can occur only by a combination of glide and climb. The stress field indicated on Fig. 9.18 shows that the set of dislocations (1) is under a compressive stress and will tend to climb up and to the right by the addition of vacancies. The set of dislocations (2) is under a tensile stress and will tend to climb down and to the right by emission of vacancies. Thus by a combination of climb and glide the boundary can move as a whole and the vacancies created at one set of dislocations are absorbed by the other. Only short-range diffusion will be required and the process will be favoured by high temperatures.

Apart from the tilt boundary discussed above, and illustrated in Fig. 9.17, the only low-angle boundary that can move entirely by glide is a cross grid of screw dislocations and in this case it is essential that the junctions do not dissociate, (see Fig. 7.17). In general, for stress induced boundary movement, some diffusion is required otherwise the boundary will break up as when a polygonised structure is deformed at low temperatures.

Movement of boundaries, in the absence of an external stress occurs during recovery and recrystallisation and requires diffusion. The principal features involved are: (a) reduction in the energy of the existing boundaries by migration to a low-energy position, as in the

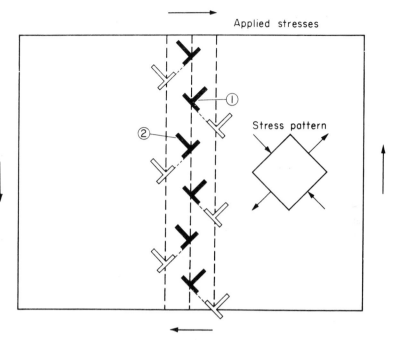

Applied stresses

Stress pattern

FIG. 9.18. Stress-induced movement of a tilt boundary containing edge dislocations with mutually perpendicular glide planes. (After READ (1953), *Dislocations in Crystals*, McGraw-Hill; from AMELINCKX and DEKEYSER, *Solid State Physics*, **18,** 325, 1958.)

first stages of recovery; (b) rotation of the crystals to reduce the angle of misorientation, thus increasing the spacing of dislocations in the boundary and reducing the energy per unit area of the boundary; and (c) movement of high-angle grain boundaries during recrystallisation and grain growth. The latter process involves an atomic rearrangement across the boundary by diffusion of atoms on a crystal of one orientation to take up positions on a crystal of a new orientation.

## 9.7 Other Dislocation Boundaries

Brief reference has aleady been made to dislocations in *deformation twin boundaries* and Fig. 6.8 illustrates the mechanism of growth of a $\{112\}$ $\langle 111 \rangle$ twin in a body-centred cubic metal by the movement of a glissile twin boundary consisting of an array of $\frac{1}{6}\langle 111 \rangle$ partial dislocations. The crystallography of $\{112\}$ $\langle 111 \rangle$ twinning in body-centred cubic metals is particulary simple and the shear displacements and atomic movements involved can be achieved by simple dislocation movements. In general, as for example in close-packed hexagonal metals, the atom movements in deformation twinning are much more complex and the dislocation configurations required to produce the observed shear displacements are correspondingly complex.

*Marternsitic transformations* produce changes in shape of a crystal which are similar to those produced by deformation twinning. The transformation from one phase to the other occurs by a shear-type process and no diffusion is involved so that the chemical composition of the two phases is the same. The changes in shape and crystal structure are usually very complex. Although it is clear that the interfaces between the martensitic transformed phase and the parent untransformed phase will involve arrays of dislocations an adequate description of these arrays has been achieved for only one or two special cases and even these are beyond the scope of this book.

However, it is appropriate to consider some aspects of the interfaces between two phases of different chemical composition and structure since they play an important part in determining the microstructure and properties of two-phase alloys. Growth of one phase with respect to the other occurs by movement of the interfaces which in turn requires diffusion of atoms across the interface. Three types of interface are possible: (a) *coherent*, (b) *semi-coherent*, and (c) *incoherent*. A coherent interface occurs between two phases in which the plane of atoms at the interface is common to the crystal structure of both phases. Thus they are likely to be found in two-phase alloys in which (i) the two phases have the same crystal structure and crystallographic orientation along with closely matched lattice parameters, for example one face-centred cubic phase embedded in another face-centred cubic phase (see section 10.6), and (ii) the two phases have different crystal structures which have a plane in common. The best example of the second type of interface occurs between face-centred cubic and close-packed hexagonal structures in which a {111} plane of the former is parallel to the (0001) basal plane of the latter. If the two phases have indentical lattice parameters it is possible for the coherent interface to be of infinite length, but this is most unlikely. Any difference in the lattice parameters will result in the development of elastic strains in the phases called *accommodation* or *coherency strains*. These will increase with the extent of the interface and eventually the coherency strains will be so large that they cannot be accommodated and this leads to the formation of a semi-coherent interface. Coherent interfaces are usually restricted to very small precipitates and small islands of a semi-coherent interface.

A semi- or partially coherent boundary is closely analogous to a low-angle boundary. The structure and formation of the boundary can be understood by reference to Fig. 9.19 which represents a section through such a boundary between two phases with atomic spacing $a_1$ and $a_2$. Because $a_1 \neq a_2$ the atoms across the boundary cannot be in perfect registry. When $a_1 - a_2$ is small matching of the boundary can be achieved (Fig. 9.19b), but elastic coherency strains are produced and the dimensions of the boundary will be limited. These strains can be accommodated by the introduction of extra planes of atoms in the top half of the crystal (Fig. 9.19c). This is equivalent to the formation of an array of edge dislocations spaced $a_1 a_2 / a_1 - a_2$ apart. Thus, a semi-coherent boundary consists of an array of dislocations separated by islands of coherent boundary. Matching of the two phases in Fig. 9.19 will also involve accommodation in directions normal to the plane of the diagram and in general the semi-coherent boundary will consist of a planar array of two or more sets of parallel or non-parallel dislocations. An example of interface dislocations on precipitates is shown in Fig. 9.20. The mechanism of formation of the network is not known, but it is clear that the large coherency

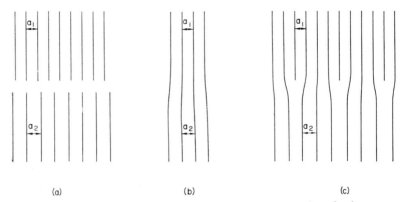

(a)                                    (b)                                    (c)

FIG. 9.19. Diagrammatic representation of a coherent and semi-coherent
interface (see text).

strains set up in the early stages of precipitation will be sufficient
to nucleate dislocations which could well be slip dislocations of the
matrix or precipitate. The stress field, strain energy, movement and
other properties of semi-coherent boundaries will depend on the type
of dislocations present in the boundary in a similar way to ordinary
dislocation boundaries described previously.

The incoherent interphase boundary is analogous to the high-angle
grain boundary and occurs when there is no simple fit between the
lattices of the two phases.

A completely different kind of dislocation array which forms during plastic deformation is the dislocation *pile-up*. Thus, consider a
dislocation source which emits a series of dislocations all lying in
the same slip plane, Fig. 9.21. Eventually the leading dislocation
will meet a barrier such as a grain boundary or sessile dislocation
configuration and further expansion of the loop will be prevented.
The dislocations emitted from the source will then pile-up against
the barrier. The strain fields of the dislocations in the pile-up will
interact elastically and the spacing of the dislocations will depend on
the applied shear stress $\tau_0$ and the type of dislocation. The distribution
of dislocations in a pile-up has been calculated by Eshelby *et al.* (1951).
For a simple pile-up of $(n-1)$ like dislocations on a single slip plane

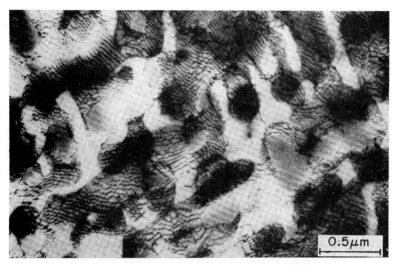

FIG. 9.20. Well-developed networks of interfacial dislocations formed during precipitation in a copper–nickel–iron alloy. (Courtesy KAINUMA and WATANABE.)

along the positive $x$-axis the number of dislocations in a slip plane, length $L$ is

$$n = \frac{L\tau_0}{2A}, \qquad (9.19)$$

where $A = A_s = Gb/2\pi$ for screw dislocations and $A = A_e = Gb/2\pi(1-\nu)$ for edge dislocations. The position of the $i$th dislocation is

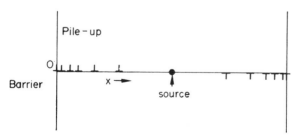

FIG. 9.21. Linear arrays of edge dislocations piled-up against barriers.

given by

$$x_i = \frac{A\pi^2}{8n\tau_0}(i-1)^2. \qquad (9.20)$$

There are two important aspects of pile-ups which are evident from this analysis. The pile-up exerts a large stress magnification at the head of the pile-up such that the stress on the leading dislocation is

$$\tau = n\tau_0 \qquad (9.21)$$

and the existence of the pile-up produces a back stress on the dislocation source given by

$$\tau_0 = \frac{2An}{L}. \qquad (9.22)$$

This stress will resist the formation of dislocation loops at the source and the expansion of existing loops.

Dislocation pile-ups have been observed many times using transmission electron microscopy. Most pile-ups will be made up of dislocations with an edge component to the Burgers vector since screw dislocations can cross slip out of the slip plane.

*Further Reading*

AMELINCKX, S. and DEKEYSER, W. (1959) "The structure and properties of grain boundaries", *Solid State Physics*, **8**, 325.

BALL, C. J. and HIRSCH, P. B. (1955) "Surface distribution of dislocations in metals", *Phil. Mag.* **46**, 1343.

BOLLMAN, W. (1970) *Crystal Defects and Crystalline Interfaces*, Springer-Verlag.

CHRISTIAN, J. W. (1965) *The Theory of Transformations in Metals and Alloys*, Pergamon Press.

ESHELBY, J. D., FRANK, F. C. and NABARRO, F. R. N. (1961) "The equilibrium of linear arrays of dislocations", *Phil. Mag.* **42**, 351.

FRANK, F. C. (1950) *Conference on Plastic Deformation of Crystalline Solids*, p. 150, Carnegie Institute of Tech. and Office of Naval Research.

FRANK, F. C. (1955) "Hexagonal networks of dislocations", *Defects in Crystalline Solids*, p. 159, Phys. Soc. London.

HU, H. (1964) "Electron transmission study of rolled and annealed silicon iron crystals", *Trans. Metall. Soc. A.I.M.E.* **230**, 572.

KEH, A. S. and WEISSMANN, S. (1963) "Deformation substructures in body-centred cubic metals", *Electron Microscopy and Strength of Crystals*, p. 231, Wiley.

LI, J. C. M. (1960) "Interaction of parallel edge dislocations with a tilt dislocation wall", *Acta Metall.* **8**, 296.

LI, J. C. M. (1963) "Theory of strengthening by dislocation groupings", *Electron Microscopy and Strength of Crystals*, p. 713, Wiley.

MARCINKOWSKI, M. J. (1972) "Dislocation behaviour and contrast effects associated with grain boundaries and related internal boundaries", *Electron Microscopy and Structure of Materials*, p. 382. University of California Press.

McLEAN, D. (1962) *Mechanical Properties of Metals*, Wiley.

McLEAN, D. (1957) *Grain Boundaries in Metals*, Clarendon Press.

MYKURA, H. (1966) *Surfaces and Interfaces*, Routledge & Kegan Paul.

READ, W. T. and SHOCKLEY, W. (1952) "Dislocation models of grain boundaries", *Imperfections in Nearly Perfect Crystals*, p. 352, Wiley.

READ, W. T. (1953) *Dislocations in Crystals*, McGraw-Hill, New York. "Recrystallisation, grain growth and textures" (1966), *American Society of Metals*, Cleveland, Ohio, U.S.A.

SCHOBER, T. and BALLUFFI, R. W. (1970) "Quantitative observation of misfit dislocation arrays in low and high angle twist grain boundaries", *Phil. Mag.* **21**, 109.

VAN DER MERWE, J. H. (1963) "Crystal interfaces", *J. Appl. Phys.* **34**, 117.

WASHBURN, J. and PARKER, E. R. (1952) *Trans. Amer. Inst. Min. (Metall.) Engrs*, **194**, 1076.

WAYMAN, C. M. (1964) *Introduction to Crystallography of Martensitic Transformations*, Mcmillan.

CHAPTER 10

# Strength of Crystals

## 10.1 Introduction

In Chapter 1 it was shown that the theoretical shear strength of a
perfect lattice is many orders of magnitude greater than the observed
critical shear of real crystals which contain dislocations. In this
next chapter the factors affecting the strength of crystals are considered
as an introduction to the way that an understanding of the properties
of dislocations can be used to interpret the properties of crystalline
solids.

Apart from effects associated with diffusion, all plastic deformation
occurs by the glide of dislocations and hence the critical shear stress
for the onset of plastic deformation is the stress required to move
dislocations. This is measured usually by a tensile test in which the
specimen is strained at a *constant rate* and the load on the specimen
is measured simultaneously with the extension. Typical stress-strain
curves are shown in Fig. 10.1. Each curve has a linear region $OE$ in
which the specimen strains elastically, obeying Hooke's law, i.e.
ratio of stress to strain is a constant. The point $E$ at which the curve
deviates from linearity represents the onset of plastic deformation. Figure 10.1(a) is typical of many materials which deform homogeneously:
the stress increases uniformly with strain. Fig. 10.1(b) is typical of
many body-centred cubic polycrystalline metals which initially
deform heterogeneously to $x$ per cent strain and then homogeneously.
The curve can be divided into four parts: (A) pre-yield microstrain,

(B) yield drop, (C) yield propagation and (D) uniform hardening. The shape of the stress-strain is sensitive to temperature, strain rate, grain size and composition. Figure 10.1(c) is typical of face-centred cubic single crystals and high purity body-centred cubic single crystals. The curve can be divided into three parts: stage I or easy glide, stage II or linear hardening and stage III which is approximately

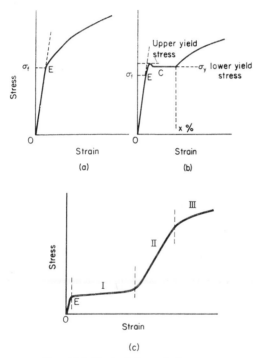

FIG. 10.1. Typical stress-strain curves.

parabolic hardening. The length of stage I and the onset of stage III are sensitive to temperature, composition and crystal dimensions whereas stage II is insensitive to these parameters. Polycrystalline face-centred cubic metals (Fig. 10.1(a)) do not show an easy glide stage and deform primarily in a way equivalent to stage III in the single crystal deformation. The stress at $E$ will be referred to as the flow stress after zero plastic strain $\sigma_{f_0}$ and the stress at $C$ as the lower yield stress or yield stress $\sigma_y$.

The applied stress required to move a dislocation in an otherwise perfect lattice depends on the binding forces beetwen atoms and is called the *Peierls stress* or *Peierls–Nabarro stress*. The simplest case is a lattice containing identical atoms. However, in the more general case the lattice may be (i) a homogeneous solid solution of one element in another, (ii) an ordered array of two or more sets of atoms forming a *superlattice*, or (iii) a lattice of positively and negatively charged ions, as in sodium chloride. There are two ways in which additional impurities in the crystal can cause an increase in the stress to move dislocations. Firstly, by arranging themselves preferentially around the dislocation to relax the large elastic strains close to the dislocation. Then the dislocation can move only by breaking away from the "atmosphere" of impurities, a process called *unpinning* or *unlocking*, or by dragging the impurities along as it moves. The force required will depend on the strength of the binding between the dislocation and the impurity atoms. Secondly, by forming clusters or precipitates in the lattice which are barriers to moving dislocations. Before the dislocations can move an appreciable distance they will be held up at the barriers and an additional force will be required for further movement. The effective strength of the barrier depends on the nature and distribution of the precipitates.

The extra dislocations introduced by strain also contribute to the strength of the crystal due to the mutual interaction between dislocations. Crystals harden progressively as straining proceeds, and the process is called *work hardening* or *strain hardening*. Theories of strain hardening attempt to explain, in terms of dislocations, the form of the stress–strain curve. Many theories have been proposed and new theories are produced year by year as more experimental observations are made and theoretical appreciation is obtained of the phenomena.

To predict the work-hardening behaviour it is essential to know how the dislocation density and distribution change with plastic strain. Thin film electron microscope observations in the past few years have shown that these parameters are sensitive to such variables as crystal structure, stacking fault energy, temperature and strain rate of deformation and it is not surprising therefore that there is no unified theory of work hardening.

## 10.2 Peierls Stress

The Peierls stress is a direct consequence of the periodic structure of a crystal lattice and depends sensitively on the exact form of the force–distance relation between individual atoms. For this reason alone the evaluation of the Peierls stress is difficult and no entirely satisfactory treatment is available. A qualitative account of Peierls stress will be given to bring out some of the important aspects.

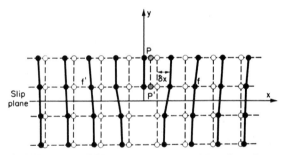

FIG. 10.2. Displacement of atoms at an edge dislocation. Open and full circles represent the atom positions before and after the extra half plane is inserted.

When an extra half plane of atoms is inserted in a lattice to simulate the formation of an edge dislocation the atoms above and below the slip plane are displaced from their equilibrium positions in the perfect lattice. This is illustrated in Fig. 10.2; the amount of the displacement $\delta x$ from the equilibrium positions decreases away from the core of the dislocation because the atoms behave as elastic rather than rigid spheres (cf. strain as a function of distance using isotropic elasticity theory). The *width w of a dislocation* is defined as the distance along the glide plane in the glide direction over which the displacement of atoms is greater than half maximum displacement, i.e. if $b$ is the magnitude of the Burgers vector of the dislocation, the maximum displacement of the atoms above the glide plane in Fig. 10.2 is $\pm b/2$ and hence $w$ is $-b/4 \leqslant \delta x \leqslant b/4$. The width will be small when the atoms are "soft" and can accommodate a considerable strain *(narrow dislocations)* and large when the atoms are "hard" *(wide dislo-*

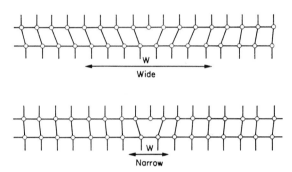

Fig. 10.3. Wide and narrow edge dislocations. (From Cottrell (1957), *The Properties of Materials at High Rates of Strain*, Inst. Mech. Eng., London.)

*cations)*; see Fig. 10.3. Estimates of $w$ depend on the form of the force–displacement relation and number of results have been quoted in the literature. The value probably lies between 1 and 10 atom spacings, but there are no experimental results to confirm this.

Any atom, $f$, or row of atoms parallel to the dislocation line, will be subjected to two principal forces, one due to the elastic stress field resulting from the introduction of the extra half plane and tending to increase $\delta x \to \pm b/2$, and the other due to the displacement of the atoms from equilibrium positions relative to surrounding atoms tending to decrease $\delta x \to 0$. Since the atoms are symmetrically arranged around the dislocation there will be a row of atoms $f'$ on the opposite side of the extra half plane under equal and opposite forces. Thus the dislocation has a system of balanced forces acting on it and is in a position of equilibrium. When the extra half plane is displaced slightly from its equilibrium position to $pp'$ the forces become slightly unbalanced and an external shear stress is required to maintain the dislocation in this position. The force required is calculated from the change in the misfit energy resulting from the displacement. The total misfit energy is obtained from a summation over all atoms displaced. To a first approximation this will be zero since, considering rows $f$ and $f'$, a displacement of $f$ in the $x$-direction will increase the misfit energy, whereas a displacement of $f'$ in the same direction will decrease the misfit energy. The difference in misfit energy arises because the work done in moving $f$ against the attractive forces between atoms is not exactly the same as the work gained as $f'$ moves with the attractive forces closer to the equilibrium position. The difference depends on the form of the force–separation relation. The maximum restraining force, i.e. the force required to move the dislocation, can be evaluated by finding the maximum rate of change in misfit energy. The simplest estimate, due to Peierls (1940) and Nabarro (1947), uses the sinusoidal force displacement relation described in section 1.3, i.e.

$$\tau = \frac{b}{a} \frac{G}{2\pi} \sin\left(\frac{2\pi x}{b}\right). \tag{10.1}$$

It follows that the restoring force is periodic. The maximum value represents the Peierls stress which for a sinusoidal relation is given approximately by

$$\tau_p \simeq 2G \exp\left(\frac{-2\pi w}{b}\right) \tag{10.2}$$

and in this analysis $w = a/(1-v)$. Since the width $w$ of the dislocation is in the exponential term the Peierls stress will be sensitive to the atom positions at the centre of the dislocation and in particular to the value of $b/a$. Taking $w = 3b$, it is immediately clear that $\tau$ is many orders of magnitude less than the theoretical shear stress (section 1.3). It cannot be over-emphasised that relation 10.2 was determined from a particular force–separation relation which has limited validity only. It may be assumed that the general form of the Peierls stress equation will contain a term $w$ which will depend on the particular force–displacement curve chosen. In spite of this

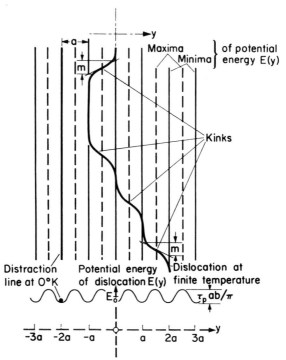

FIG. 10.4. The potential energy surface of a dislocation line due to the Peierls stress $\tau_p$. The figure is not drawn to scale, since in reality $E_0 \gg (\tau_p^0 ab/\pi)$ and $m \gg a$. (From SEEGER, DONTH and PFAFF, *Disc. Faraday Soc.* **23**, 19, 1957.)

uncertainty a number of features of the Peierls model are generally accepted: (a) in most crystals the Peierls stress is small, particularly, for example, in face-centred cubic metals; (b) in crystals with a significant Peierls stress the dislocations will tend to lie along specific crystallographic directions, as in Fig. 8.7; (c) in crystals with narrow dislocations the Peierls stress may contribute significantly to the variation of the flow stress with temperature.

To understand these features it is more convenient to consider the potential energy of a dislocation as a function of its position in the crystal. Following Seeger, the potential energy surface of a dislocation line can be represented by Fig. 10.4. $E_0$ is the energy per unit length of dislocation line and will be given approximately by equations (4.9) and (4.10). The periodic variation of the potential energy of the dislocation due to the position of the dislocation in the lattice has an amplitude $\tau_p ab/\pi \ll E_0$ and a period $a$ related to the spacing of the close-packed planes and also the Burgers vector.

Consider a length of dislocation $AB$ in Fig. 10.5(a) lying in a position of minimum energy along a close-packed direction in the lattice and suppose that an applied stress is tending to move it in a direction perpendicular to itself. If the dislocation behaves as a rigid rod a stress equal to the Peierls stress will be required to move it over the potential barrier to the next equilibrium position, $CD$.

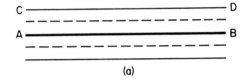

(a)

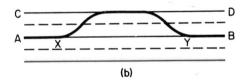

(b)

Fig. 10.5. Seeger's dislocation mechanism. (a) Dislocation in position of minimum energy. (b) Bulge in dislocations.

This type of behaviour is expected for dislocations in a crystal at 0 K. At finite temperatures the dislocation will no longer lie in only one valley of its potential energy surface but will contain kinks (Fig. 10.4), i.e. it will change from one valley to a neighbouring one.

The shape and length $m$ of the kink will depend on the magnitude of the energy barrier between one equilibrium position and the next. The minimum energy form of the dislocation at the kink will be a curved line (Fig. 10.6). The form of the curve is determined by a balance between two opposing factors: (i) the dislocation tends to lie as much as possible in the position of minimum energy (this factor alone would give the shape shown by curve *A* (Fig. 10.6); (ii) the dislocation tends to reduce its energy by being as short as possible— which favours the straight line shape *B*.

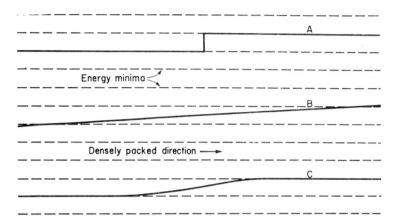

FIG. 10.6. Shape of dislocations running almost parallel to a densely packed direction. The energy per unit length of the dislocation is a minimum along the dashed lines and varies periodically at right angles to the lines. The shape of the dislocation (curve *C*) is somewhere between the extremes *A* and *B*. (From READ, (1953) *Dislocations in Crystals*, McGraw-Hill)

If the energy hump is a large fraction of the average energy $E_0$, then factor (i) above dominates and the kink is short and has a relatively high energy. As the energy hump decreases the kinks become larger and the dislocation approaches the straight line shape *B* and kink energy decreases.

If a stress $\tau < \tau_p$ is applied to a dislocation line containing kinks (Fig. 10.4) it can more forward by two processes: (1) sideways movement of the kinks which will require very small stresses, because the potential barriers opposing motion in directions parallel to the close-packed directions are small, and (2) formation of a small *bulge*, as a result of thermal fluctuation, which can then spread sideways (Fig. 10.5).

## 10.3 Interaction between Point Defects
## and Dislocations

Each point defect, i.e. vacancy or interstitial atom, substitutional or interstitial impurity atom produces a stress field in the surrounding lattice which will interact with the elastic stress field of the dislocations. If the defect diffuses to the dislocation or the dislocation moves to the defect the strain energy of the system may be lowered. Additional work will be required to separate the defect and this will result in an increase in the stress to move dislocations. The crystal will be stronger. The simplest example of this effect is the accommodation of an over-sized atom at an edge dislocation. The hydrostatic compressive stresses around an atom will be relaxed if the atom is situated in the dilated region below the extra half plane of the edge dislocation and, there-fore, the atom will be attracted to the dilated region and repelled from the compressed region.

The interaction energy can be determined as follows. Consider an atom of natural radius $a(1+\varepsilon)$ resting in a hole of natural radius $a$ (cf. section 8.4) in an isotropic material. If $\varepsilon \neq 0$ the atom will produce a symmetrical hydrostatic distortion of the surrounding matrix. The interaction energy is the work done against the local stress field in producing this distortion

$$U_i = p\Delta V, \qquad (10.3)$$

where $p = -\frac{1}{3}(\sigma_x+\sigma_y+\sigma_z)$ is the hydrostatic pressure of a stress field at some point; $\sigma_x$, $\sigma_y$ and $\sigma_z$ are the normal stress components, and $\Delta V = 4\pi\varepsilon a^3$ is the change in volume of the hole. Thus

$$U_i = -\tfrac{4}{3}\pi\varepsilon a^3(\sigma_x+\sigma_y+\sigma_z). \qquad (10.4)$$

For an atom situated at a point with rectangular coordinates $x$, $y$, $z$ from an edge dislocation lying along the $z$-axis, and with Burgers vector along the $x$-axis, the interaction can be calculated directly using equations (4.6) and 4.7)

$$U_i = \frac{4}{3} \frac{(1+\nu)}{(1-v)} \frac{Gb\varepsilon a^3 y}{(x^2+y^2)}, \qquad (10.5)$$

or in cylindrical coordinates $r$, $\theta$,

$$U_i = \frac{4}{3}\frac{(1+\nu)}{(1-\nu)}\frac{Gb\varepsilon a^3 \sin\theta}{r},$$  (10.6)

since $r = (x^2+y^2)^{\frac{1}{2}}$ and $\sin\theta = y/(x^2+y^2)^{\frac{1}{2}}$.

$U_i$ will have a maximum positive value when the solute atom is situated immediately above the slip plane in the region of the extra half plane ($\theta = \frac{1}{2}\pi$) as close as possible to the centre of the dislocation, and maximum negative value when the solute atom is immediately below the extra half plane ($\theta = \frac{3}{2}\pi$). The latter represents the site of maximum relaxation at the dislocation and the difference in energy between an atom in this position and the same atom situated at a large distance from the dislocation is the *binding energy* of the defect to the dislocation.

Several modifications are necessary in applying this approach to defects in real crystals since the assumptions made in the analysis have only limited validity. These assumptions are:

(a) The solute atom is completely rigid. If the solute atom has the same elastic properties as the matrix additional strain energy will be introduced due to elastic deformation of the solute atom. Taking this effect into account Bilby (1950) obtains

$$U_i = 4Gb\varepsilon a^3 \frac{\sin\theta}{r}.$$  (10.7)

(b) The matrix behaves as an isotropic elastic material. In practice, the matrix will be crystalline and have a periodic stress field. This may have a significant effect on the interaction energy particularly close to the dislocation core.

(c) The strain field around the dislocation and the defect does not affect the electron distribution in the lattice.

(d) The dislocation is not dissociated into partial dislocations and a stacking fault.

The original calculation of $U_i$ by Cottrell was directed towards an understanding of the yield behaviour of iron and, in particular, the interaction between carbon atoms and dislocations in iron. In the case of interaction with an edge dislocation the simple model above is a good representation of the physical situation and gives a realistic binding energy $\sim 0.2$ aJ. However, a similar calculation for a pure screw dislocation using the same approximations would give an interaction energy of zero, because the field of a screw dislocation has no hydrostatic component. This is unlikely and the difficulty is resolved by considering the position of the interstitial atoms in the lattice. For example consider the carbon and nitrogen atoms in the body-centred cubic iron lattice. The most favourable site is of the

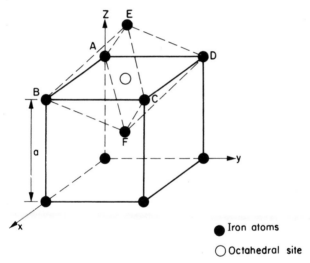

● Iron atoms

○ Octahedral site

FIG. 10.7. Octahedral interstitial site in a body-centred cubic cell.

type $\frac{1}{2},\frac{1}{2},0$, i.e. in the centre of the cube face, as illustrated in Fig. 10.7. Since $AC = BD = a\sqrt{2}$ and $EF = a$, the introduction of a spherical atom with a diameter larger than $(a-2r)$ where $r$ is the radius of an iron atom, will produce a tetragonal distortion by displacing atoms $E$ and $F$ outwards. Thus an atom introduced into such a site will produce both a hydrostatic and a shear stress field which will interact with pure screw dislocations as well as edge dislocations.

A difference in the elastic properties of the defect and matrix will modify further the elastic interaction, and thereby affect the interaction energy. When the volume change due to introduction of the atom is large, as in the case of interstitial carbon in iron, the effect will be relatively small. However, for substitutional solute atoms in a face-centred cubic crystal the effect may be significant, since the volume change is relatively small.

Vacancies and interstitial matrix atoms also interact elastically with a dislocation. The interaction with an interstitial atom will be similar to the interaction with an interstitial impurity atom, but the volume change is normally much larger. A dilational strain field is formed round a vacancy and hence a vacancy is attracted to the compressive region above the slip plane of an edge dislocation.

So far only elastic interactions have been considered. Additional contributions to the interaction energy result from the following electrical and chemical effects.

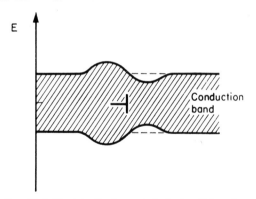

FIG. 10.8. Electric dipole created at edge dislocation.

(a) The local density changes around an edge dislocation, due to the compressive and tensile stresses associated with the extra half plane, may produce a rearrangement of the conduction electrons around the dislocation, as illustrated in Fig. 10.8. In the dilated region below the extra half plane an excess of electrons causes a net negative charge and in the denser region there is a net positive charge. The charge distribution along the dislocation is essentially an electric dipole which can interact with a point defect having a different electronic charge than a matrix atom at the same site, e.g. solute atoms (interstitial or substitutional) having a different valency, and vacancies. This effect may be important in some metals, but it is unlikely to represent more than about 10 per cent of the total interaction energy.

(b) In polar crystals such as NaCl, KCl, LiF, and AgCl, the lattice consists of differently charged ions which interact with each other electrostatically. Each ion occupies an equilibrium position in the electrostatic field of the other ions. The removal of one ion results in the formation of a *positive ion vacancy* or a *negative ion vacancy* which will interact strongly with, for example, jogs in dislocations which in these crystals will carry a net positive or negative charge as illustrated in Fig. 6.11. In this case, the electrical interaction is greater than the elastic interaction.

(c) When a unit dislocation dissociates into partial dislocations a stacking fault is formed between the partials, as described in section 5.3. This affects the periodic arrangement of the lattice and, in a face-centred cubic metal, the region close to the fault will have a close-packed hexagonal stacking. The difference in structure may give rise to different thermochemical properties such that, for example, the solubility of solute in the face-centred cubic and close-packed lattices is different. This will result in an interaction between the extended dislocation and the solute. This type of interaction has been called *chemical interaction*.

## 10.4 Locking and Friction Strengthening

The interaction energy between a defect and a dislocation depends on the position of the defect relative to the dislocation. To achieve "equilibrium" conditions the defect will diffuse to the position of maximum relaxation in the vicinity of the dislocation. Before the dislocation can move a force will be required to overcome the interaction forces between the defect and dislocation (section 10.5). The dislocation is said to be *locked* by the impurities. Many of the interaction processes described in section 10.3 can produce this effect. Once the dislocation has been separated from the defects its movement is unaffected by the locking process. Locking can be "reintroduced" by allowing the defects to diffuse to the dislocation again and this is the basis of *strain ageing*.

The movement of an unlocked dislocation is controlled by the so-called *friction stresses*, $\sigma_i$, which have many forms and are additive in their effect on the strength of a crystal. The friction stress is due to the interaction of the moving dislocation with for example (a) the crystal lattice i.e. Peierls force (section 10.2), (b) other dislocations section 10.8, (c) individual solute atoms, i.e. substitutional hardening (section 10.6), (d) vacancies and interstitial atoms as, for example, in irradiation and quench hardening, (e) clusters or precipitates of solute atoms in precipitation hardening (section 10.6), and (f) clusters of vacancies or interstitials. For a crystal under an applied stress $\sigma_{appl}$, the effective stress on the dislocation is $\sigma_{eff} = \sigma_{appl} - \sigma_i$.

## 10.5 Unlocking Stress

The magnitude of the stress required to separate a dislocation from defects will depend on the number and distribution of defects at the dislocation and the way in which the separation occurs. These two aspects are considered in terms of the separation of an edge dislocation in iron from carbon impurities. Similar arguments will apply to other systems since the interaction energy is of a similar form. The approach used below is simplified considerably, as will be obvious when reference is made to the list of assumptions in section 10.3.

Consider an edge dislocation in a crystal which contains impurity atoms having an interaction energy with the dislocation of the form

$$U_{(i)} = \frac{A \sin \theta}{r}. \tag{10.8}$$

Lines of equal interaction energy around an edge dislocation have been plotted in Fig. 10.9. When the defects can diffuse they will tend

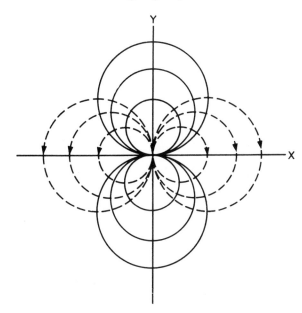

Fɪɢ. 10.9. Equipotential lines (full lines) for the elastic interaction potential given by equation (10.8), between an edge dislocation along the $z$-axis with Burgers vector parallel to the $x$-axis and solute atoms. Broken lines are lines of flow for solute atoms migrating to the dislocation. (After Cᴏᴛᴛʀᴇʟʟ and Bɪʟʙʏ, *Proc. Phys. Soc.* A, **62**, 49. 1949.)

to lower their energy by moving to the dilated region below the extra half plane and the dotted lines in Fig. 10.9 represent the lines of flow. The latter are drawn perpendicular to the lines of equal interaction energy and indicate the path the defects will take to the dislocation in the absence of diffusion parallel to the dislocation line.

When one atom has diffused to the position of maximum relaxation the interaction between the dislocation and a second defect will be modified. For any given concentration of defects in the matrix an equilibrium distribution will be established around the dislocation. Above a critical concentration two additional effects have been considered: (a) formation of a row of carbon atoms and (b) formation of definite precipitate particles (Fig. 10.10). Further discussion will

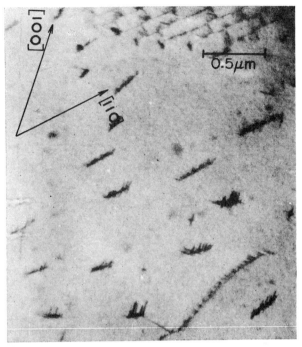

Fig. 10.10. Transmission electron micrograph of carbide precipitate particles formed along dislocations in iron. The particles are in the form of platelets and are viewed edge-on. (From Hull and Mogford, *Phil. Mag.* **6**, 535, 1961.)

be limited to (a) since this produces maximum locking of the dislocation.

Consider a condensed row of carbon atoms lying in the position of maximum binding at an edge dislocation as illustrated in Fig. 10.11. (Note, the number of atomic sites at the position of maximum binding is approximately equal to $N$, the dislocation density and, therefore, the atomic concentration of carbon atoms required to produce condensed rows on all the dislocations will be $\sim Nb^2$ where $b$ is the atomic spacing. Taking $N = 10^6$ dislocations mm$^{-2}$ and $b = 0.3$ nm gives a concentration of carbon atoms of only $10^{-5}$ at. per cent.) An applied stress will tend to separate the dislocation, along

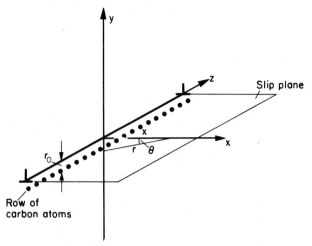

F<small>IG</small>. 10.11. Diagrammatic representation of a row of carbon atoms lying in the position of maximum binding at an edge dislocation. An applied shear stress will cause the dislocation to separate from the carbon atoms by gliding in the slip plane to position $x$.

its slip plane, from the row of carbon atoms. Using the interaction equation (10.8), the interaction energy at a displacement $x$, measured in the slip plane, from the carbon atoms is

$$U_{(i)} = -\frac{Ar_0}{r^2} = -\frac{Ar_0}{x^2+r_0^2}.$$

(10.9)

The force per atom plane intersected by the dislocation required to separate the dislocation to a distance $x$ is

$$F_{(x)} = \frac{\partial U_{(x)}}{\partial x} = \frac{2Ar_0x}{(x^2+r_0^2)^2}.$$

(10.10)

This is illustrated in Fig. 10.12. The separation for the maximum value of $F_x$ is obtained by differentiating and equating to zero, thus

$$x = \frac{r_0}{\sqrt{3}}$$

(10.11)

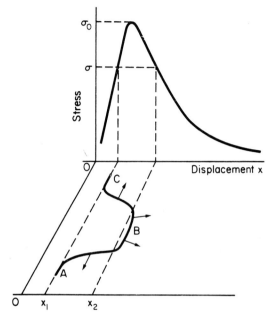

FIG. 10.12. Separation of a dislocation from a row of condensed carbon atoms. Initially the dislocation lies along the line $x = 0$. Under the applied stress $\sigma$ it moves forward to the position of stable equilibrium $x_1$. To break away it must reach the position of unstable equilibriujm $x_2$. *ABC* represents a loop of dislocation, formed by a thermal stress fluctuation, in the process of breaking away. (From COTTRELL (1957), *Properties of Materials at High Rates of Strain*, Instn. Mech. Eng., London.)

and the corresponding value of $F_{(x)}$ per atom plane

$$F_{(x)\,\text{max}} = \frac{3\sqrt{(3)}\,A}{8r_0^2}\,. \tag{10.12}$$

The critical stress, per unit length of dislocation, required to separate the dislocation from the row of carbon atoms is, therefore,

$$\sigma_0 = \frac{3\sqrt{(3)}\,A}{8r_0^2 b^2}\,. \tag{10.13}$$

When realistic values for $A$ are used it is found that $\sigma_0$ is close to the stress to start plastic deformation at temperatures near 0 K. However, the observed stress decreases with increasing temperature and this has been explained by taking account of the effect of thermal activation (Cottrell and Bilby, 1949).

In determining the critical stress it was assumed that the dislocation remained parallel to the row of carbon atoms all along its length. If the dislocation line is flexible it is possible that local fluctuations in thermal energy can cause the dislocation to separate from the carbon atoms by forming a loop of dislocation line as illustrated in Fig. 10.12. The stable position of the dislocation in the absence of an applied stress is along $O$–$O$. When a stress is applied ($\sigma < \sigma_0$) the dislocation will move to $x_1$ which will be a position of stable equilibrium due to the balance between the interaction stress and the applied stress. The position $x_2$ is that of unstable equilibrium beyond which the applied stress always exceeds the effective internal stress pulling the dislocation back to its anchorage. It is proposed that the loop extends beyond $x_2$ and therefore it will tend to expand under the applied stress and pull the remainder of the dislocation from the anchorage by an unzipping process.

It is expected that the flow stress associated with dislocation locking will increase rapidly with decreasing temperature. The absolute magnitude of these stresses and the effect on the yield and flow stress of crystals is a matter for speculation. It is known that the yield stress of body-centred cubic metals is extremely temperature sensitive at low temperatures, but as already suggested, the Peierls stress will probably make an important contribution to this dependence. Other features, such as dislocation velocity, multiplication rate and impurity interaction with moving dislocations may be important also.

## 10.6 Strengthening by Precipitate Particles

When a crystal of element $A$ contains atoms of another element $B$ in supersaturated solid solution, the latter will tend to precipitate in the solvent metal as particles of either pure $B$ or a compound of $A$ and $B$. The formation of the second phase occurs by nucleation and growth of the precipitate particles as a result of diffusion. At low temperatures diffusion is very slow and the supersaturated solution is frozen in. One example is the solution of carbon in iron referred to in section 10·3 in connection with dislocation locking. Another example is the solution of copper in aluminium. A section of the aluminium–copper phase diagram is shown in Fig. 10.13.

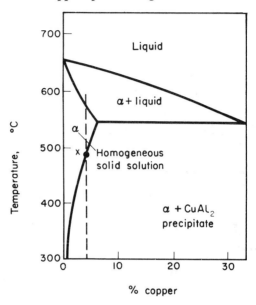

Fig. 10.13. Section of the aluminium–copper equilibrium diagram.

An alloy containing 4 per cent copper which is heated to 550°C will be a *homogeneous solid solution*. When the alloy is cooled slowly the second phase will start to precipitate out at the temperature indicated by point $x$ and at 20°C the alloy will consist of large $CuAl_2$ precipitates in an aluminium-rich matrix. However, if the alloy is quenched from 550°C a supersaturated solid solution is obtained. On subsequent heating to, say, 150°C the copper atoms come out of solution to produce *precipitates* which change in size, morphology and composition with time. Two important forms of the precipitate which are common to many systems are *coherent* and *incoherent*.

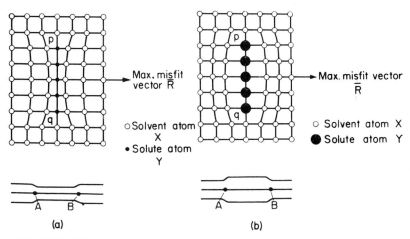

FIG. 10.14. Schematic representation of zones which give rise to coherency strains. (a) For small solute atoms. (b) For large solute atoms. (From THOMAS (1963), *Electron Microscopy and Strength of Crystals*, p. 793, Interscience.)

A precipitate or zone with a *coherent interface* (see section 9.7) is illustrated in Fig. 10.14. A layer of $Y$ atoms has displaced $X$ atoms along a plane represented by $p$–$q$. Since the $Y$ atoms are smaller than the $X$ atoms the lattice around the platelet will have to accommodate the shape change by elastic strain, in a similar way to the elastic strain round an individual solute atom. The elastic strain around the coherent precipitates can be relieved in two ways: (a) creation of dislocations in the matrix, as described in section 8.4, and formation of a dislocation interface to produce a *semi coherent boundary*; (b) bulk diffusion; when this occurs the interface is normally a high angle boundary and is therefore *incoherent*.

Substitutional solute atoms can produce three basic hardening effects due to: (a) substitutional solid solution, (b) coherent precipitates or zones, (c) precipitates. In each case, a moving dislocation has to circumvent or overcome the resistance provided by these barriers. As precipitation from supersaturated solid solution proceeds the sequence (a) → (b) → (c) occurs and the hardness of the alloy chan-

ges accordingly as demonstrated in Fig. 10.15. After quenching the
solid solution is harder than the pure metal and on heating or ageing
at 150°C the hardness increases due to the formation of coherent
zones (this is the basis of age-hardening in, for example, commercial
aluminium base alloys). Peak hardness corresponds to the position of
optimum size, distribution and coherency strains of the precipitates.

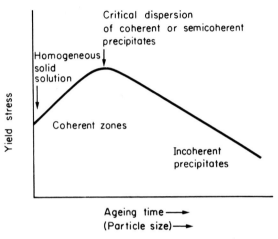

FIG. 10.15. Variation of yield stress with ageing time typical of an age-
hardening aluminium alloy.

The hardness drops due to formation of larger semi-coherent and
incoherent precipitates.

The interpretation of the strengthening by solute atoms and precipitates is usually based on theories due to Mott and Nabarro (1948).
It is assumed that resistance to dislocation movement is due to the
elastic strain field round a spherical particle radius $a$ (section 10.3)

$$\frac{\varepsilon a^3}{r^3} \, (r > a), \tag{10.14}$$

where $\varepsilon$ is the misfit parameter. Modifications are necessary to the
theory to include the different elastic modulus of the precipitate and
the matrix, the particle morphology, the exact nature of the coherency

strain, and the way the dislocation overcomes or cuts through the barriers; these aspects are discussed in detail by Kelly and Nicholson (1963).

Consider a perfectly straight dislocation line lying in a crystal with randomly distributed solute atoms, as illustrated in Fig. 10.16. When the dislocation is close to a solute atom its strain field will interact

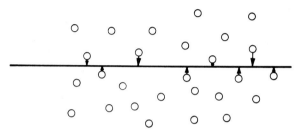

FIG. 10.16. Straight dislocation in a crystal with randomly distributed solute atoms.

with that of the solute atom and the dislocation will be attracted or repelled according to the sign of the dislocation. Providing the dislocation remains straight, there will be no net force on the dislocation since the algebraic sum of all the interaction energies will be zero, and the solute atom strain fields will provide no resistance to the dislocation. In practice, the dislocation line is *flexible* and will take up a lower energy position by bending round regions of large interaction energy. For a local stress at a solute atom or particle the maximum bending that the stress can sustain is given by equation (4.19)

$$\varrho \simeq \frac{Gb}{2\tau_0}.$$

It follows that the position of the dislocation, and hence the type of interaction, will depend on the average spacing $\varLambda$ of the particles.

If a crystal contains an atomic concentration of solute atoms, $c$, these may exist as a large number of closely spaced individual atoms or as a relatively small number of widely spaced particles. Depending

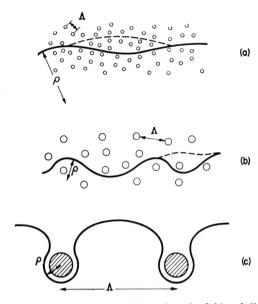

FIG. 10.17. Movement of flexible dislocations in fields of dispersed obstacles. The circles enclose regions of high energy for the dislocation, i.e. zones or precipitates and their associated strain fields. The new position of the dislocation after a unit movement is represented by the broken line. (a) Very small zones or individual solute atoms, $\Lambda \ll \varrho$. (b) Intermediate sized particles with $\Lambda \simeq \varrho$. (c) Large precipitates $\Lambda \gg \varrho$; loops of dislocation form round the precipitates.

on the size and spacing of the particles three situations may be considered, see Fig. 10.17.

### (a) VERY FINELY DISPERSED PARTICLES OR INDIVIDUAL SOLUTE ATOMS

The wavelength of the internal stress field, i.e. $\Lambda$, is very small and for individual atoms is $b/c^{1/3}$ where $b$ is the interatomic spacing. The local stress fields are not sufficient to bend the dislocation round each individual particle and

$$\Lambda \ll \varrho. \tag{10.15}$$

The dislocation therefore over-rides partially the strain field of the particles, but since it is flexible it takes up, under a given shear stress, a position where there is a net positive interaction energy.

Mott and Nabarro made two calculations for the flow stress $\tau_0$ by a summation of the forces on the dislocation. The first calculation gave

$$\tau_0 = G\varepsilon^2 c \qquad (10.16)$$

which was in agreement with some experimental results, and a later estimation gave

$$\tau_0 = 2\cdot5G\varepsilon^{4/3}c \qquad (10.17)$$

for values of $c$ between $10^{-2}$ and $10^{-3}$. Both these relations predict that solid solution hardening is directly proportional to the solute concentration and this is in agreement with many experimental results.

(b) COHERENT OR SEMI-COHERENT PRECIPITATES, $\approx$ 10 nm APART

The dislocations can bend round the particles such that

$$\Lambda \simeq \varrho \qquad (10.18)$$

as illustrated in Fig. 10.17(b). The loops of dislocation formed can move independently of each other. Glide occurs by each dislocation loop overcoming the interaction energy of the particle. This has normally been assumed to be entirely due to the elastic strain field, but an important contribution is almost certainly provided by the work done in shearing the particle because new particle-matrix interfaces are produced.

Neglecting the work done in the cutting process, the flow stress is the average internal stress and, according to Mott and Nabarro, is given by

$$\tau_0 = 2G\varepsilon c \qquad (10.19)$$

and is independent of the spacing $\Lambda$ of the particles providing the above description is applicable. When the crystal is in this condition it is at maximum hardness (see Fig. 10.15). The critical spacing of the precipitates can be obtained from equation (4.19) since

$$\varLambda \simeq \frac{Gb}{2\tau_0}. \tag{10.20}$$

Therefore, substituting for $\tau_0$ in equation (10.19)

$$\varLambda_c \simeq \frac{b}{4\varepsilon c}. \tag{10.21}$$

Taking $\varepsilon = 0\cdot2$, $c \simeq 0\cdot02$ gives $\varLambda_c \simeq 60b$.

### (c) Large, Widely Separated Particles Typical of Over-aged Alloys

The mean distance between particles is much larger than the limiting radius of the dislocation, thus

$$\varLambda \gg \varrho. \tag{10.22}$$

The crystal is soft and the dislocation can bow out between the particles. The flow stress is that required to bend the dislocations to a radius $\frac{1}{2}\varLambda$, i.e.

$$\tau \simeq \frac{Gb}{\varLambda}. \tag{10.23}$$

As each dislocation bows round the precipitate it will leave a loop of dislocation, as illustrated. This will result in an increase in flow stress with increasing strain, due to the back stress resulting from the dislocation rings around the precipitate.

The strengthening mechanisms described in sections 10.3 to 10.6 all involve the presence of either impurity atoms or alloying elements. The list of mechanisms is far from complete. Another important group of strengthening mechanisms is associated with the resistance to dislocation motion produced by the presence of long-and short range order which may modify the core structure of dislocations or provide obstacles to moving dislocations.

## 10.7 Plastic Strain and Yield Drop

In this section the relation between dislocation movement and plastic strain will be described and related to the plastic instability which produces the yield drop. Following Gilman (1961), consider a crystal (Fig. 10.18) containing edge dislocations which have moved

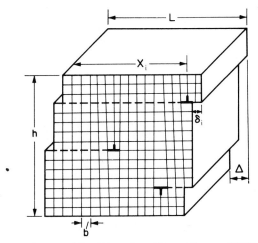

FIG. 10.18 Strain caused by dislocations (From GILMAN (1961), *Mechanical Behaviour of Materials at Elevated Temperatures*, p. 17. McGraw-Hill.)

various distances through a unit cube of the crystal. The total displacement of the top of the cube with respect to the bottom is $\Delta$. Each dislocation contributes a small displacement $\delta_i$. When a dislocation moves completely across the crystal it causes a displacement $b$. Since $b$ is very small compared with $L$ or $h$, the displacement $\delta_i$ for a dislocation at an intermediate position between $x_i = 0$ and $x_i = L$ will be proportional to the fractional displacement $x_i/L$. Therefore

$$\delta_i = \frac{x_i b}{L}, \tag{10.24}$$

then

$$\Delta = \sum \delta_i = \frac{b}{L} \sum_{1}^{N} x_i, \tag{10.25}$$

where $N$ is the total number of dislocations that have moved. The macroscopic shear strain $\varepsilon$ is given by

$$\varepsilon = \frac{\Delta}{h} = \frac{b}{hL}\sum_{1}^{N} x_i. \tag{10.26}$$

The sum can be replaced by the product of the number of dislocations moving $N$, and the average distance moved $\bar{x}$. Since $h$ and $L$ are unity,

$$\varepsilon = bN\bar{x}. \tag{10.27}$$

The strain rate will be

$$\frac{d\varepsilon}{dt} = \dot{\varepsilon} = bN\bar{v}, \tag{10.28}$$

where $\bar{v}$ is the average dislocation velocity.

The same argument can be used for screw dislocations and for a complete loop of dislocation line the macroscopic strain is proportional to the area swept out by the loop, $\varepsilon = bA$, and for $N$ loops ,

$$\varepsilon = bNA. \tag{10.29}$$

Similarly,

$$\dot{\varepsilon} = b(N_s\bar{v}_s + N_e\bar{v}_e) \tag{10.30}$$

assuming only pure screw and pure edge dislocations are present.

Measurement of a stress–strain curve involves an interaction between a specimen and some kind of machine. Therefore, the machine characteristics must be taken into account in interpreting the observations. For a specimen tested in an elastic, hard-beam machine a displacement in the specimen is equal to the displacement of the crosshead less the elastic displacement in the system. This can be understood by reference to Fig. 10.19 using an approach described by Johnston and Gilman (1959). A specimen is being tested in a uniaxial tensile machine, but the approach is equally applicable to other types of test. The elasticity of the machine and specimen is represented by an

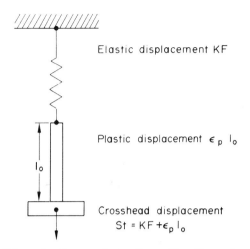

FIG. 10.19. Schematic diagram of a tensile machine. The spring represents the elastic propesties of the machine and specimen. (After JOHNSTON and GILMAN, *J. Appl. Phys.* **30**, 129, 1959).

imaginary spring. The crosshead moves at a constant speed $S = dl/dt$ so that the cross head displacement at time $t$ is $St$. The total elastic displacement of the spring is $KF$ where $F$ is the applied force and $K$ the spring constant. The plastic displacement of the specimen is $\varepsilon_p l_0$ where $\varepsilon_p$ is the plastic strain and $l_0$ is the original gauge length. Thus

$$St = KF + \varepsilon_p l_0. \qquad (10.31)$$

The plastic strain of the specimen is

$$\varepsilon_p = \frac{St - KF}{l_0} \qquad (10.32)$$

and the plastic strain rate is

$$\dot{\varepsilon}_p = \frac{S - K\dfrac{dF}{dt}}{l_0}. \qquad (10.33)$$

Taking the resolved shear stress $\tau$ as $F/2A_0$, where $A_0$ is the original cross-sectional area of the specimen, gives

$$\frac{d\tau}{dt} = \frac{S - \dot\varepsilon_p l_0}{2A_0 K}. \qquad (10.34)$$

Since $S = dl/dt$ the measured hardening rate

$$\frac{d\tau}{dl} = \frac{1}{2A_0 K}\left(1 - \frac{\dot\varepsilon_p l_0}{S}\right) \qquad (10.35)$$

can be seen to be dependent on the elastic properties of the machine and specimen and the instantaneous plastic strain rate of the specimen.

The shape of the stress–strain curve given by equation (10.35) can be related to the dislocation behaviour through the plastic strain rate term $\dot\varepsilon_p$ using equation (10.28). However, since both $N$ and $\bar v$ will vary with stress and strain it is necessary to know the variation of both before any predictions can be made. This information is only available in isolated cases. Johnston (1962) has reviewed the effects of all the machine and specimen dislocation variables on the stress–strain curve and some of his results are illustrated in Fig. 10.20. The calculations were based on data obtained from LiF crystals in which the measured dislocation density increases with strain in the early stages as

$$N \approx 10^9 \varepsilon \qquad (10.36)$$

and the dislocation velocity can be related to the applied shear stress through a relation of the type (3.3a) viz.

$$\bar v = (\tau/\tau_0)^m \qquad (10.37)$$

where $m = 16.5$ for LiF.

Figure 10.20(a) shows the effect of changing the initial density of mobile dislocations from $N_0$ from 0 to $5 \times 10^6$ dislocations cm$^{-2}$. The line $OE$ represents the situation where there is no dislocation movement $\dot\varepsilon_p = bN\bar v = 0$ in equation (10.35), i.e. completely elastic behaviour, $d\tau/dl = \frac{1}{2}A_0 K$. The curves show that a sharp yield drop is obtained for low values of $N_0$ and that the yield drop decreases as

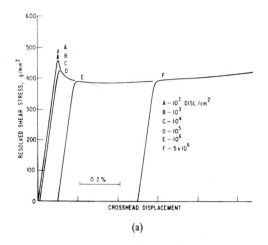

(a)

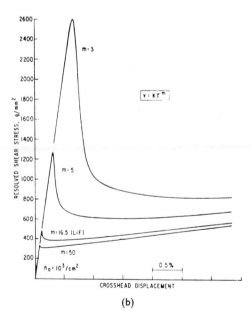

(b)

FIG. 10.20. (a) Effect of initial density of mobile dislocations on the yield point. (b) Effect of changing the stress dependence of dislocation velocity on the yield point. (After JOHNSTON, *J. Appl. Phys.* **33**, 2716, 1962).

$N_0$ increases. The curves in Fig. 10.20(a) have been displaced from the origin for convenience. The yield drop can now be interpreted in the following way. Suppose that a crystal containing a fairly low density of dislocations which are free to glide is strained using a constant crosshead speed. At low stresses the dislocations cannot move fast enough to produce a sufficient strain in the specimen and therefore the stress rises. As the stress rises, dislocations multiply rapidly and they move faster. The stress stops rising, $d\tau/dl = 0$, when $bN\bar{v} = S/l_0$ (equation (10.35)), i.e. the strain rate of the crystal equals the applied strain rate. However, multiplication continues with increasing strain, producing more than enough dislocations $bN\bar{v} > S/l_0$. The stress, therefore, drops until the dislocation motion becomes so slow that the strain rate of the crystal equals the applied strain rate again.

Figure 10.20b shows the calculated stress–strain curves for different values of the parameter $m$ in equation (10.37). The results in Fig. 3.11 indicate that the stress dependence of dislocation velocity varies considerably from one material to another. The shape of the calculated stress–strain curves show a strong dependence on $m$.

In general three conditions must be satisfied for the occurrence of a yield drop. (1) The initial dislocation density must be small, (2) the dislocation velocity must not increase too rapidly with increasing stress, (3) the dislocations must multiply rapidly. The first, and most important, condition can be achieved very simply by "locking" the dislocations by one of the methods described in section 10.4. In lithium fluoride and body-centred cubic metals locking is obtained readily by impurity atom interaction. In face-centred cubic metals locking can be produced by alloying and by irradiation with energetic particles.

In single crystals yielding starts by the formation of a few isolated slip bands, probably at a region of local stress concentration, due to the release of "locked" dislocations or the nucleation of fresh dislocations. The dislocations can multiply by the multiple cross glide and Frank–Read mechanisms to form broad slip bands, and by the formation of new slip bands. In most single crystals the multiplication rate is not very great and the yield drop is fairly small. However, it can be very large, and the extreme case is the yield drop obtained in *whisker* crystals. These are extremely small crystals $\sim 1$ $\mu$m diameter which can be produced free from dislocations. The stress–strain curve of a copper whisker is shown in Fig. 10.21. The maximum stress $\tau_{max}$ is close to the theoretical strength and dislocations are nucleated

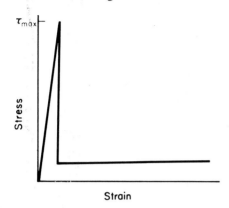

FIG. 10.21. Stress–strain curve of a copper whisker (see Brenner, 1958).

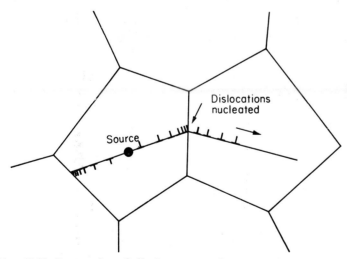

FIG. 10.22. Propagation of slip from one grain to an adjacent grain. Dislocation sources in the new grains close to the grain boundary are activated by the stress field around the dislocation pile-up.

homogeneously. However, once dislocations have been produced they multiply very rapidly and the stress drops to normal values.

In polycrystalline specimens, pre-yield microstrain is confined to isolated grains. This is due to the barriers to slip provided by grain boundaries. It is usually assumed that local regions of high stress concentration, such as small inclusions and grain boundary triple-point junctions, initiate slip in favourably orientated grains. Consider a grain in which slip has been initiated; the dislocations will be confined to a narrow band and will propagate until they meet the grain boundary. As the stress increases this process will occur in other grains. A stage is reached at which the stress at the end of a slip band at a grain boundary is sufficient to initiate slip in the next grain as illustrated in Fig. 10.22. For simplicity it is assumed that the dislocations have a pure edge character and lie on a single slip plane. In practice they will have a mixed character and may be distributed on a number of slip planes. The dislocations in the next grain are produced either by nucleation in the crystal close to the boundary, or by the unlocking of existing dislocations, due to the stress concentration at the head of the pile-up. The new slip band can itself nucleate slip in the next grain and, at a citical stress, the process rapidly spreads across the specimen.

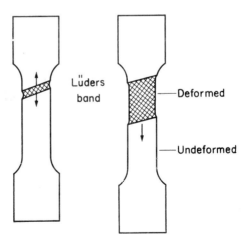

FIG. 10.23. Lüders band propagation.

This process represents a very rapid dislocation multiplication and can result in a large yield drop. The initial zone of deformation is called a *Lüders band* and the boundary between the band and undeformed parts of the crystal is called the *Lüders front* as illustrated in Fig. 10.23. The Lüders front propagates down the specimen at approximately constant stress until the whole of the specimen is deformed. The state of strain and the dislocation distribution is then approximately homogeneous throughout the specimen. In most specimens more than one Lüders band forms and they grow towards each other.

## 10.8 Theories of Flow Stress

The stress at which plastic flow starts is called the *flow stress* (see section 10.1). In well-annealed single crystals, the flow stress will be the critical resolved shear stress, but in more general terms it is represented by any point on the stress–strain curve. For any given state of plastic strain there is a critical stress $\tau_f$ required to produce further deformation. Since deformation occurs by the movement of dislocations the critical stress is determined by the stress required to move dislocations through other dislocations and obstacles in the material. The flow stress is normally considered to be made up of a component $\tau_G$ which is independent of temperature apart from the variation of the elastic modulus $G$ with temperature, and a component $\tau_S$ which increases with decreasing temperature. Thus,

$$\tau = \tau_G + \tau_S. \tag{10.38}$$

The particular dislocation arrangements which may contribute to $\tau_G$ and $\tau_S$ are discussed later in this section.

It follows that, depending on the type of obstacles present, the flow stress will vary with temperature and strain rate. A simple analysis (following Seeger, 1957) will be used to illustrate the variation with temperature. Consider a crystal at a particular strain, containing $N$ mobile dislocations per unit volume held up at energy barriers, which can be overcome with the aid of thermal energy and the applied stress. To overcome the barriers each dislocation must acquire an energy $U_b$

over a length $l$. If the dislocation has to move through a distance $d$ in this process, the "*activation volume*" will be

$$V = b\,d\,l. \tag{10.39}$$

Since the energy $U_b$ can be provided by the thermal energy and by the work done by the applied stress, the activation energy can be written

$$U = U_b - V\tau, \tag{10.40}$$

$U_b$ will consist of two parts. Firstly, the energy required to push the dislocation through the internal stress field in the lattice. In the absence of effects other than dislocations, this is usually attributed to long range elastic interaction between dislocations and is given by $V\tau_G$. Secondly, the local energy barrier $U_0$ associated with the actual intersection of dislocations

$$U_b = U_0 + V\tau_G. \tag{10.41}$$

Thus
$$U = U_0 - V(\tau - \tau_G). \tag{10.42}$$

If the dislocation sweeps out an average area $A$ after it overcomes a barrier the strain rate will be given by the Arrhenius equation

$$\dot\varepsilon = bANv_0 \exp\left\{-\frac{U}{kT}\right\}, \tag{10.43}$$

where $v_0$ is the frequency with which the dislocation tries to overcome the barrier, which will depend on the nature of the obstacle and the way it is overcome. $v_0$ has an upper limit equal to the Debye frequency $\approx 5\times10^{12}$ sec$^{-1}$. Assuming that $d$ and $l$ are independent of $(\tau-\tau_G)$, Seeger (1957) obtained the variation of flow stress with temperature by combining equations (10.42) and (10.43)

$$\tau = \tau_G \quad \text{when} \quad T \geqslant T_0,$$

$$\tau = \tau_G + \tau_S, \tag{10.44}$$

$$= \tau_G + \frac{U_0 - kT\ln\left(\dfrac{NAbv_0}{\dot\varepsilon}\right)}{V}$$

when $T \leqslant T_0$,

where

$$T_0 = \frac{U_0}{k \ln \left( \dfrac{NAbv_0}{\varepsilon} \right)}.$$  (10.45)

Thus for $T \geqslant T_0$ the flow stress will be practically independent of temperature, and for $T \leqslant T_0$ the flow stress will increase with decreasing temperature. The predicted temperature dependence is illustrated in Fig. 10.24. It is emphasised that this approach assumes that there is only one thermally activated process that is rate controlling throughout the entire temperature range.

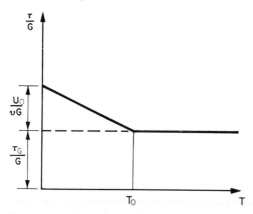

FIG. 10.24. Temperature dependence of the flow stress, $\tau$, according to equation (10.44) (From Seeger (1957), *Dislocations and Mechanical Properties of Crystals*, p. 243, Wiley.)

In practice there are numerous types of barrier to dislocation motion arising from the presence of dislocations in the lattice. Each type of barrier will provide a different kind of resistance to motion. Many of these barriers have already been described and they may be summarised as follows:

(a) Elastic interaction with stress fields of individual dislocations. Two main contributions can be distinguished: (i) interaction with dislocations parallel to the moving dislocations and (ii) interaction with dislocations which intersect the slip plane, i.e. *forest dislocations*.

(b) Elastic interaction with stress fields of piled-up groups of dislocations which form in the lattice at sessile dislocations.

(c) Elastic interaction with stress fields of high-energy dislocation networks and tangles.

(d) Interaction with "debris" produced by dislocation movement such as point defects and dislocation loops.

The *work-hardening behaviour* of a material will depend on the type, distribution and number of barriers which form during straining. Many models and theories have been proposed.

*Further Reading*

ARDLEY, G. W. (1955) "Effect of ordering on the strength of $Cu_3Au$", *Acta Metall.* **3**, 525.

ARGON, A. S. (1972) "Thermally activated motion of dislocations through random localized obstacles," *Phil. Mag.* **25**, 1053.

BASINSKI, Z. S. (1959) "Thermally activated glide in face-centred cubic metals", *Phil. Mag.* **4**, 393.

BASINSKI, Z. S. and WEINBERG, F. (1967) (Eds.) *Deformation of Crystalline Solids, Can. J. Phys.*

BILBY, B. A. (1950) "On the interaction of solute atoms and dislocations", *Proc. Phys. Soc.* A, **63**, 191.

BRENNER, S. S. (1958) "Properties of whiskers", *Growth and Perfection of Crystals*, p. 157, Wiley.

BROWN, N. (1959) "Yield point of a superlattice", *Phil. Mag.* **4**, 693.

BULLOUGH, R. and NEWMAN, R. C. (1962) "The interaction of vacancies with dislocations", *Phil. Mag.* **7**, 529.

CLAREBROUGH, L. M. and HARGREAVES, M. E. (1959) "Work hardening of metals", *Progress in Metal Physics*, Vol. 8, p. 1, Pergamon, London.

COCKHARDT, A. W., SCHOECK, G. and WIEDERSICH, H. (1955) "Interaction between dislocations and interstitial atoms" *Acta Metall.* **3**, 533.

COTTRELL, A. H. (1954) "Interaction of dislocations and solute atoms", *Relation of Properties to Microstructure*, p. 131, Amer. Soc. Metals, Cleveland, Ohio, U.S.A.

COTTRELL, A. H. (1957) "Deformation of solids at high rates of strain", *The Properties of Materials at High Rates of Strain*, Instn. Mech. Eng., London.

COTTRELL, A. H. and BILBY, B. A. (1949) *Proc. Phys. Soc.* A, **62**, 49.

"Dislocations in solids" (1964) *Disc. Faraday Soc.* **38**,

FISCHER, J. C. (1954) "Strength of solid solution alloys" *Acta Metall.* **2**, 9.

FLEISCHER, R. L. (1961) "Solution hardening", *Acta Metall.* **9**, 996.
FLEISCHER, R. L. (1963) "Substitutional solution hardening", *Acta Metall.* **11**, 203.
FRIEDEL, J. (1964) *Dislocations*, Pergamon Press.
GILMAN, J. J. (1962) "Debris mechanism of work hardening", *J. Appl. Phys.* **33**, 2703.
GILMAN, J. J. (1969) *Micromechanics of Flow in Solids*, McGraw-Hill.
GUYOT, P. and DORN, J. E. (1967) "A critical review of the Peierls mechanism", *Can. J. Phys.* **45**, 983.
HIRSCH, P. B. (1964) "A theory of linear strain hardening", *Disc. Faraday Soc.* **38**, 111.
HIRSCH, P. B. and HUMPHREYS, F. J. (1970) "The deformation of single crystals of copper and copper-zinc alloys containing alumina particles", *Proc. Roy. Soc.* A, **318**, 45.
HIRTH, J. P. and LOTHE, J. (1968) *Theory of Dislocations*, McGraw-Hill.
JOHNSTON, W. G. (1962) "Yield points and delay times in single crystals", *J. Appl. Phys.* **33**, 2716.
JOHNSTON, W. G. and GILMAN, J. J. (1958) "Dislocation velocities, dislocation densities and plastic flow in lithium fluoride crystals", *J. Appl. Phys.* **30**, 129.
JOSSANG, T., SKYLSTAD, K. and LOTHE, J. (1963) "Theory of thermal activation of dislocations over the Peierls barrier", *Relation Between Structure and Strength in Metals and Alloys*, H.M.S.O., London.
KEH, A. S. and WEISSMANN, S. (1963) "Deformation sub-structures in body-centred cubic metals", *Electron Microscopy and Strength of Crystals*, p. 231, Interscience, New York.
KELLY, A. and NICHOLSON, R. B. (1963) "Precipitation hardening", *Prog. Mat. Sci.* **10**, 148.
KUHLMANN-WILSDORF, D. (1962) "A new theory of work hardening", *Trans. Metall. Soc. A.I.M.E.* **224**, 1047.
LI, J. C. M. (1963) "Theory of strengthening by dislocation groupings", *Electron Microscopy and Strength of Crystals*, p. 713, Wiley.
MADER, S., SEEGER, A. and THEERINGER, H. M. (1963) *Relation Between Structure and Strength in Metals and Alloys*, H.M.S.O., London.
MCLEAN, D. (1962) *Mechanical Properties of Metals*, Wiley.
MOTT, N. F. (1952) "Mechanical strength and creep in metals", *Imperfections in Nearly Perfect Crystals*, p. 173, Wiley.
MOTT, N. F. (1960) "The work hardening of metals", *Trans. Metall. Soc., A.I.M.E.* **218**, 962.
MOTT, N. F. and NABARRO, F. R. N. (1948) *Strength of Solids*, p. 1, Phys. Soc, London.
NABARRO, F. R. N. (1947) "Dislocations in a simple cubic lattice", *Proc. Phys. Soc.* **59**, 256.
NABARRO, F. R. N. (1967) *The Theory of Crystal Dislocations*, Oxford University Press.
NABARRO, F. R. N., BASINSKI, Z. S. and HOLT, D. B. (1964) "The plasticity of pure single crystals", *Adv. Physics*, **13**, 193.
OROWAN, E. (1947) "Discussion", *Symposium on Internal Stresses*, p. 451, Inst. Metals, London.

PEIERLS, R. (1940) "The size of a dislocation", *Proc. Phys. Soc.* **52**, 34.
ROSENFIELD, A. R., HAHN, G. T., BEMENT, A. L. and JAFFEE, R. L. (1968) *Dislocation Dynamics*, McGraw-Hill.
SEEGER, A. (1957) "Glide and work hardening in face-centred cubic and hexagonal close-packed metals", *Dislocations and Mechanical Properties of Crystals*, p. 243, Wiley.
TAYLOR, G. I. (1934) "Mechanism of plastic deformation of crystals", *Proc. Roy. Soc.* A, **145**, 362.

# The SI System of Units

*Base-units*

| | |
|---|---|
| metre (m) | — length |
| kilogram (kg) | — mass |
| second (s) | — time |
| ampere (A) | — electric current |
| kelvin (K) | — thermodynamic temperature |
| candela (cd) | — luminous intensity |

*Some derived units*

| | name of SI unit | SI base-units |
|---|---|---|
| frequency | hertz (Hz) | $1\ Hz = 1/s$ |
| force | newton (N) | $1\ N\ = 1\ kg\ m/s^2$ |
| work, energy | joule (J) | $1\ J\ \ = 1\ Nm$ |

*Multiplication factors*

| | Prefix | Symbol |
|---|---|---|
| $10^{12}$ | tera | T |
| $10^9$ | giga | G |
| $10^6$ | mega | M |
| $10^3$ | kilo | k |
| $10^{-3}$ | milli | m |
| $10^{-6}$ | micro | $\mu$ |
| $10^{-9}$ | nano | n |
| $10^{-12}$ | pico | p |
| $10^{-15}$ | femto | f |
| $10^{-18}$ | atto | a |

*Some useful conversions*

| | |
|---|---|
| 1 angstrom | $= 10^{-10}\ m = 100$ pm or 0.1 nm |
| 1 kgf | $= 9.8067\ N$ |
| 1 atm | $= 101.33\ kN/m^2$ |
| 1 torr | $= 133.32\ N/m^2$ |

| | |
|---|---|
| 1 dyne | $= 10^{-5}$ N |
| 1 dyne/cm | $= 1$ mN/m |
| 1 cal | $= 4.1868$ J |
| 1 erg | $= 10^{-7}$ J $= 0.1$ µJ |
| $10^6$ erg/cm$^{-2}$ | $= 1$ kN/m |
| 1 inch | $= 25.4$ mm |
| 1 lb | $= 0.4536$ kg |
| 1 lbf | $= 4.4482$ N |
| 1 lbf/in$^2$ | $= 6894.76$ N/m$^2$ |
| 1 lb/in | $= 0.1751$ kN/m |
| 1 eV | $= 1.6 \times 10^{-19}$ J $= 0.16$ aJ |

# Index